Our Diabetic Sons
Living And Surviving
The Severe
Complications
Of Diabetes

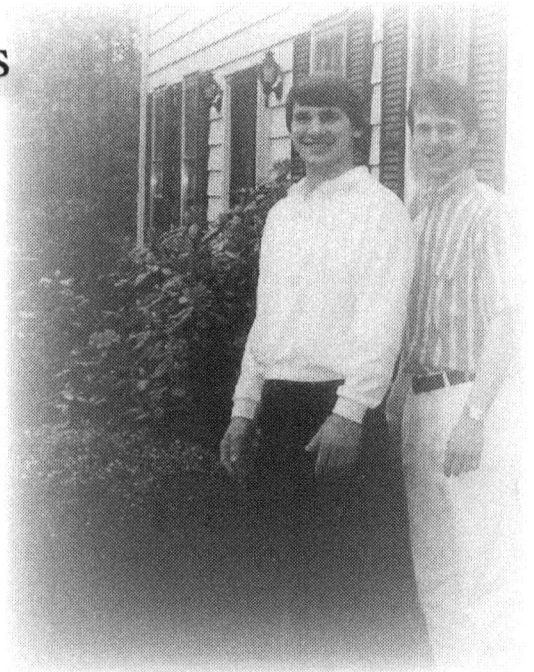

By
Martha E. Tuck

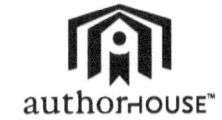

authorHOUSE™

1663 LIBERTY DRIVE, SUITE 200
BLOOMINGTON, INDIANA 47403
(800) 839-8640
WWW.AUTHORHOUSE.COM

First published by AuthorHouse 01/06/06

ISBN: 1-4208-7416-0 (sc)

Library of Congress Control Number: 2005907410

Printed in the United States of America
Bloomington, Indiana

This book is printed on acid-free paper.

TABLE OF CONTENTS

ACKNOWLEDGMENTS vii

DEDICATION ix

INTRODUCTION xi

PREFACE xvii

CHAPTER 1 DIAGNOSED – 1977 1

CHAPTER 2 DIABETES STRIKES AGAIN 7

CHAPTER 3 GOLDEN OPPORTUNITY *
HYPERGLYCEMIA 18

CHAPTER 4 NEW HORIZONS 23

CHAPTER 5 DOCTOR'S CONCERN 34

CHAPTER 6 EYE SURGERIES * DISABILITY 40

CHAPTER 7 GOOD AND BAD TIMES 48

CHAPTER 8 DIALYSIS TREATMENT * DIET 59

CHAPTER 9 WHAT IS DIALYSIS? 63

CHAPTER 10 GETTING READY FOR TRANSPLANT 69

CHAPTER 11 DISAPPOINTING NEWS 82

CHAPTER 12 PREPARING FOR TRANSPLANT 88

CHAPTER 13 TRANSPLANT 94

CHAPTER 14 ADJUSTING * HUMAN-INTEREST STORY 104

CHAPTER 15 OKT3 TREATMENT * BIOPSY * SELLING
MODIFIED 112

CHAPTER 16 URETERAL STENT * EXPLORATORY
SURGERY 121

CHAPTER 17 SCLEROTHERAPY TREATMENT *
SURGERY (BIG ONE) * TORNADO 127

CHAPTER 18 LOSING HOPE * LAURA'S INVITATION *
FRONT PAGE HEADLINE 141

CHAPTER 19 NEW YEAR * NEW BEGINNINGS 156

CHAPTER 20 ISLET CELL TRANSPLANTS *
NIGHT OF PURE HELL 167

CHAPTER 21 SECOND OPINION * A DREAM
COME TRUE.. 173

CONCLUSION 183

EPILOGUE 184

ACKNOWLEDGMENTS

I would like to give "Special Thanks" to all our family and friends that helped to give us inner strength when we needed it the most.

Also to the following for their forbearance, understanding and support during our difficult time: Transplant Doctors, Johann Jonsson, Timothy Shaver, Roslynn Manson, and the entire Transplant team and nurses at Fairfax Hospital. Transplant Coordinators: Pat DiSanto and Jade Robinson.

As well as Doctors: John C. Baldinger, Michael F. Ball, Earl P. Grober (now deceased), Michael Hardy, Mauricio D. Bas, Jr., Robert E. Greenspan, and all Personnel at the Dialysis Center. Last, but not least, to the Riverview Baptist Church for all their thoughts and prayers as they helped to pull us through.

For all those mentioned above, we thank you! We are forever, eternally grateful.

I would also like to give my humble thanks to my lovely granddaughter, Leah Schwenger, and her dear friend Helen Jaques for proof reading and editing my memoir. Leah being just eight-years-old at the time of her Uncle Doug's transplant was not aware of what all her Uncle Doug had to go through. As well as her Uncle David – she was amazed.

A "special" thank you goes to my wonderful daughter-in-law, Margie, whom was very patient with me in helping to get all my pictures placed in the right order for my book. She is a blessing!

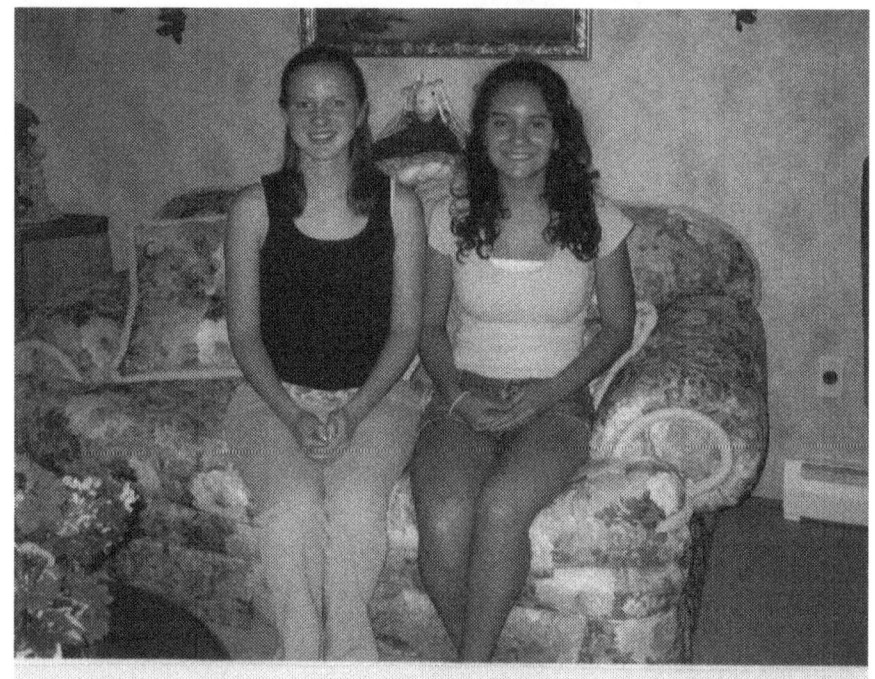

Leah & friend, Helen

DEDICATION

OUR DAUGHTER, OUR HERO

With Laura knowing and seeing the misery her younger brother, Doug, was going through while on Dialysis, she made up her mind to do something about it. Knowing in advance that he would need a kidney transplant, she did not think twice about being his donor.

For doing this Laura, your Dad and I are dedicating this book to you. "You are truly our Hero." We love you!

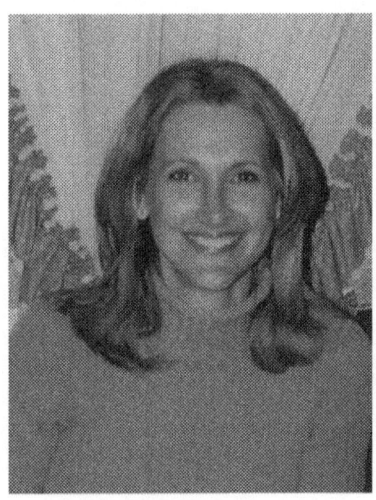

INTRODUCTION

There are 18.2 million Americans with Diabetes and over 5 million of them do not even know they have it. Diabetes contributes to the death of 213,000 Americans each year and is also a leading cause of heart disease, blindness, and kidney failure! Not to mention nerve damage and amputations as well.

What exactly is diabetes? Diabetes Mellitus, now called (Type 1), is a chronic disease characterized by inability to burn up the sugars (carbohydrates), which have been ingested. It is caused by insufficient production of insulin by the pancreas. In people with Type 1 diabetes, insulin-producing cells have been destroyed – leaving the pancreas unable to regulate blood glucose levels. Besides the presence of too much sugar and other products in the blood and urine, symptoms may include great thirst, passing large amounts of urine, loss of weight, and loss of strength.

When sugar is absorbed from the digestive tract, the blood to the body's cells carries it. Normally, with the help of insulin (a hormone made in the pancreas), the cells use sugar for energy to store for later use. But in people with diabetes, insulin is either lacking (absent or reduced) or is not effective. In either case, the cells are unable to make use of the sugar, which collects in the blood and, eventually, in the urine. Treatments for diabetes aim to keep blood-sugar levels in the near-normal range, in hopes of preventing complication. People with diabetes are born with a genetic tendency to develop the disease, but other causes also play a role.

What Is Autoimmunity? Since the late 1970's, medical researchers have recognized that diabetes is an autoimmune disease in which the body's own cells are destroyed by the immune system. The process leading to diabetes may begin years before the symptoms of the disease appear. In those people who are genetically predisposed to diabetes, the body's cytotoxic T lymphocytes begin to attack the insulin-producing beta cells, possibly mistaking certain proteins in the cells as proteins from an invading virus. Gradually, as the beta cells are destroyed, insulin production begins to taper off. When 80 to 90 percent of the beta cells are destroyed, the person is unable to produce sufficient insulin, and they very suddenly develop symptoms of diabetes.

There are two main types of diabetes: Insulin-dependent (Type 1) diabetes occurs most often in children and young adults and must be treated with insulin injections and an appropriate meal plan.

Non-insulin-dependent (Type II) diabetes occurs most often in adults over 40, especially in the obese. Treatment for non-insulin-dependent diabetes is exercise and a meal plan emphasizing weight loss. For some people, doctors may also prescribe pills that help to control blood sugar or insulin injections.

You are at an increase risk for (Type II) diabetes if you are: African American, Hispanic/Latino, Native American, Asian American or

Pacific Islander; Over age 45; under active; Overweight or obese; Someone with a family history of diabetes; A woman who has had a baby weighing more than nine pounds at birth. People with (Type II) diabetes may develop slowly and often have no symptoms, but those that do, have the same symptoms as Type 1. As well as other signs including frequent infections, blurred vision, cuts, or bruises that are slow to heal, tingling or numbness in the hands or feet, and recurring skin, gum or bladder infections.

Many people do not realize that it was not until 1922 that insulin began to be used on patients with diabetes – until that time, it was extremely rare for patients with Type1 diabetes to live more than one or two years after being diagnosed! Even though there have been great advances in improving the lives of those affected by diabetes, there still is not a cure for this devastating disease and current treatments have only limited success in controlling its devastating consequences.

Many people think that diabetes is a "mild" disease or is "cured" by insulin, but neither impression is true. While insulin is crucial to the day-to-day survival of many people, it is not a cure. People with diabetes are at risk for serious health problems (complications), which many include heart disease, stroke, kidney disease, blindness, nerve damage, and severe infection leading to gangrene and foot and leg amputations.

I consider diabetes the worse disease a person can get. It's worse than heart disease or cancer because you suffer aggravation, inconvenience, pain, and medical complications over a long period of your life, if not most of it.

What one does now is certainly a lot less primitive than it was 25 years ago. Then, most people with Type 1 diabetes would have taken one shot a day, some even with only NPH insulin. We did not ever measure blood sugar levels at home – we measured glucose levels with urine tests. Hemoglobin A1cs were not available 25 years ago, so there was no way to measure quality of control. And, of course, we did not know the long-term consequences of control because there had been no studies such as the DCCT (Diabetes control and complications trial) as there is today.

One of the hidden dangers of diabetes is hypertension (high blood pressure), which if left untreated, can lead to kidney failure. The risks for heart attacks, stroke and kidney failure are significantly greater in those who have untreated high blood pressure...especially since many of the effects of both diabetes and high blood pressure do not become apparent until it's too late!

Diabetic Nephropathy: Nearly one-third of all patients with Type 1 (insulin dependent) diabetes ultimately develop kidney failure due to diabetic nephropathy. Unlike other kidney diseases, diabetic nephropathy is silent in its early stages. Signs and symptoms of the disease, such as high blood pressure, decreased renal function, and protein in the urine, do not show up until kidney damage is advance. At this stage, when the disease is obvious, treatment is of little value, except that it may slow the rate of destruction. Ultimately, nephropathy leads to a condition known as end-stage renal disease (ESRD) for which kidney transplantation or dialysis are the only available treatments. One of the most fortunate things about your kidneys is that you really only need about 10% of their capacity. Almost 90% of their function can be lost before there are outward signs of kidney failure.

The Sacrifice: The lives of every patient's family members are affected - they can't go on vacation without arranging for dialysis at a remote location...young children often can't play after school due to their dialysis schedules...even cooking meals becomes more difficult due to the special dietary needs of dialysis patients!

Almost every one of these newly diagnosed patients face financial crisis. Some have their life savings drained because many of their treatment-related expenses are not covered by insurance. Others lose their jobs because their medical condition does not allow them to continue their line of work.

There's more to diabetes than one can ever imagine. It isn't just taking a shot. So many non-diabetics are not aware of this. Not knowing what's involved, it's hard for them to understand why one does one thing and one does another. Every diabetic is different. What one requires may not necessarily mean the other one would. It is important for people who are free of this disease to know something about it so as not to judge unfairly to those who suffer from it.

The book you're about to read is written from a mother's perspective, and is based on our family and its trials and tribulation's living with diabetes. After reading my story, I hope, I have helped others to gain knowledge on diabetes and its major complications, as well as the urgent need for donor-organ donation. I would like to think, I've succeeded in doing so...

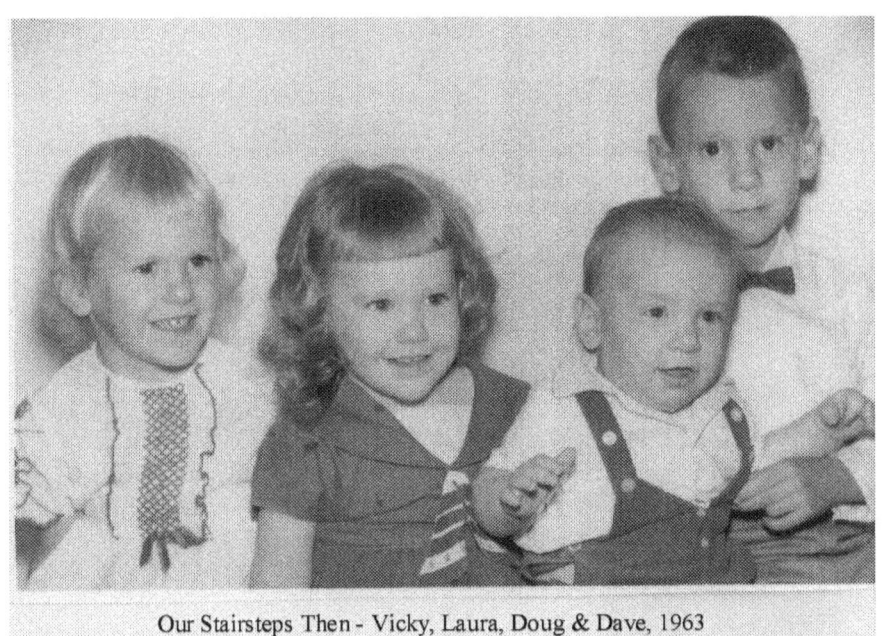

Our Stairsteps Then - Vicky, Laura, Doug & Dave, 1963

PREFACE

My story begins in 1955 in Alexandria, Virginia where Vic and I met in high school. Becoming sweethearts, we quit school to become husband and wife in January 1958. With me being 16 and Vic 17 at that time, we were somewhat more mature than most at our age. Having lived in an era when times were tough, but fun, one tends to grow up fast.

The first five years of our married life produced four children. Having out grown our two-bedroom apartment, we bought our first new home in Woodbridge, Virginia in 1963. It is located approximately twenty-five miles south of Washington, D.C.

We had four wonderful, happy, healthy children at that time. With David being almost 5, Vicky at 2 ½, Laura 17 months and Douglas 4 months – we called them our "Stair steps!" Our family life was as normal as any other in the Sixties. Although, the cost of living and housing was cheaper – with a wife and four children to support, Vic worked hard holding two jobs to help make ends meet.

We did not get out but once a year back then, and that was to celebrate our wedding anniversary. I am not complaining, though, we had Elvis and the Beatles on the music charts, a new home, job, and healthy kids. What more could one want? Life was good!

Changing Circumstances – 1977: Historians tend to concentrate on years of dramatic action, but more often than not, history is a process of slow and undramatic adjustment to changing circumstances. 1997 was such a year. We had a new President, James Earl Carter, Jr., of Georgia. We had new leaders in congress – a new speaker of the House of Representatives, Thomas P. (Tip) O'Neill, Jr., (D., Mass.), and a new majority leader of the Senate, Robert C. Byrd (D., W.Va.).

Together, they tackled the old problems of unemployment and inflation and the health, education, and welfare of the nation – with great vigor and some success, but without any spectacular results.

On August 23, 1977, our family life – like history, became a process of slow and undramatic adjustment to changing circumstances. We also had problems of unemployment, health, and welfare – with some

success, and at times without any spectacular results. The following
is such a story:

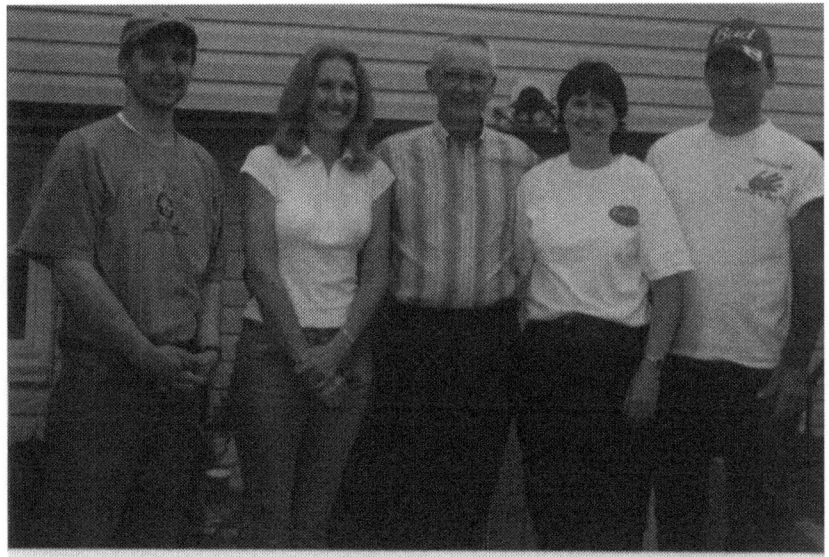

Our Stairsteps Now - David, Laura, Vicky and Doug with
their dad, Vic on Father's Day, June 20, 2004

CHAPTER 1

DIAGNOSED – 1977

The sun was shining high in a blue, cloudless sky that hot Tuesday morning on August 23, 1977. Doug, our youngest, had just been diagnosed with Juvenile Diabetes. Now called Type 1 or Insulin-Dependent Diabetes. When leaving the doctors office that morning, I felt as blue as the sky looked and the tears in my eyes clouded a bright sunny day.

Doug turned 14 the first day of spring on March 20th of that year. A few months prior to that, he began complaining with several different ailments he'd had. "My heart is beatin' so hard and fast it feels like it's comin' through my chest!" he announced one day after experiencing, a strong, rapid heartbeat. As time went on there was not a day that went by that he did not complain about something. It was either a headache, backache, or it would be some type of pain in his arms or legs. He was constantly running to the refrigerator taking doses of Pepto-Bismol, for what he called an "upset stomach".

Discussing this with my parents, my dad informed me that kids going through puberty experience "harmless" growing pains. Saying they have all kinds of unusual symptoms, which he had implied, that was probably happening to Doug.

1

With Doug's continual complaints, and with him never a sickly child, I made an appointment in mid-May to see our family doctor, John S. Greenhalgh. Having a physical and blood work done at that time, we were later told all tests came back normal. Although nothing was found wrong, neither Doug's symptoms nor his complaints lessen.

Then three months later in late August, I started seeing signs I was not used to seeing. His running to get something to drink every few minutes, and the numerous times he went running to the bathroom. However, being as active as he was in the summer's heat at the time, I overlooked it all to just that.

Searching for answers: Glancing through my medical book one evening searching for an answer due to this frequency, I came upon some of his symptoms in the diabetic section. To my surprise, he had two of the three main ones - excessive thirst and frequent urination. The third one, weight loss, was not seen at that time. Thinking it was an inheritable disease, I knew of no one on either side of our families that ever had it. After reading the article, though, I knew I should get Doug rechecked soon, if he continued having symptoms.

The following morning, I was in the process of getting ready for work as a County School Crossing Guard. While in the bathroom, Doug called for me from across the hall. "Mom, I don't feel too good," he said weakly, as he held onto his bedroom door to keep from falling. While looking at him, I knew something was terribly wrong. I could not believe what I was seeing! Our once, healthy, looking boy looked as if he had deteriorated overnight. Having lost a great amount of weight and drained of all his strength and energy, he stood slumped over with his arms hung limply by his side. His rounded cheeks had become thin, and he had dark circles under his eyes.

With this all happening overnight, I stood there looking at him and thinking he was dying from some horrible disease I knew nothing about. "Go back to bed," I told him. "I'll call the doctor when I get back from my crossing." Calling within an hour, the receptionist informed they were all booked up for the day. "Sorry," she said, when hearing his symptoms in needing to see the doctor.

Not being able to get an appointment, I discouragingly hung up the phone. Going back to Doug's room and seeing how bad he looked, I marched back to the phone and redialed again. By this time I was steaming! After all, I thought, I gave her all of Doug's symptoms. She should have known by that how sick he was! The nerve of her, I muttered to myself while dialing. "I know you told me Doug could not be seen today," I told the receptionist upon answering, "but I told you before how sick my son was." "If the doctor can not see him in the office," I snapped, "then he'll see him in the hospital! One way or another, he has to be seen today!" "All right, Mrs. Tuck," she replied with a sarcasm tone. "If you must, then bring him on in."

Doctor Greenhalgh checked Doug thoroughly that day. Also taking a urine test, and seeing his blood sugar was over 500, we were told to take Doug straight to the hospital to be admitted. "I'll call the hospital and let them know you're coming," Dr. Greenhalgh said.

Whereupon, he told us if Doug had waited another day or so to be seen, he could have gone into a coma. With tear-filled eyes when leaving the doctors office that morning, the same young receptionist that had been so uncooperative earlier that morning when I had called, smiled shyly and muttered, "I'm so sorry," as I walked out the door.

Admitted: On August 23, 1977, Doug was admitted to Potomac Hospital in Woodbridge, just a short distance from home. Having changed our lives drastically from there on out. Although we had heard of diabetes, we had no idea what all was involved. As a family, we had so much to learn.

In the hospital, they taught Doug how to give his own injections by inserting a needle into an orange. He did well, and it did not take long for him to adjust in giving his own injections. They also taught me the procedure, so I could give the injections when he came home. I did not have to do it for long, as he wanted to do it on his own. "I can do it," he'd say, with me taking more precise time than he. "See, just stick it in! It doesn't hurt!"

Needle injections were never a problem with Doug having diabetes – it was his diet. The dietician at the hospital tried to regulate the diet according to his age, weight and exercise to the amount of insulin he was taking. However, with Doug a growing teen, seeing all his food weighed and measured, as well as the amount he could eat, was quite upsetting for him. With his doctor knowing the diet was not working that well with him, suggested letting him eat the amount that satisfied

4

him by readjusting the insulin with his food intake. This new approach made a much happier Doug.

Doug was always a very active child in keeping busy most of the time, so the five days he was in the hospital was very hard on him. With his days restless ones, I tried staying with him for as long as I could during the day. I was totally exhausted both physically and mentally by days end. Before ever reaching the door when I arrived from the hospital each evening, I would hear the phone ringing. It was Doug, wanting to talk, and who needed answers to try to understand all the changes his body was now undertaking – crying at times.

Between my trips back and forth to the hospital each day, I had my family at home to care for too. Doing this and worrying about Doug, added a lot of extra stress on me. Not to mention having to learn all about insulin, needles, injections, urine checking, high and low sugar, diet, and the weighing and measuring of food. I was going through the same thing as Doug – confused, trying to comprehend it all.

Glucose Monitoring: Having been referred to a Diabetic Doctor, we were informed about the blood-glucose monitoring system and how the monitors are of great asset to a diabetic. By pricking one's finger, we were told, with a small needle and placing it in a blood glucose meter would give the diabetic his or her blood sugar reading. With a normal glucose-sugar reference reading being 65-109.

In 1977, the blood monitors were fairly new to the market. They could be purchased through your doctor only, with some insurance companies covering some, or none of the cost. With the monitors quite expensive, our insurance did not cover such an item; therefore, Doug had to rely testing his blood sugar readings using the urine (diastix) strips.

By dipping urine on the diastix strip and comparing result by the color chart on the bottle, would give the diabetic his or her blood sugar reading. The diastix and clinistix were two special urine-testing kits on the market, which at that time, was the only source for diabetics to monitor their blood sugar.

Doug (12), Laura(13), David (17) and Vicky (15). This picture was taken before Doug was diagnosed with diabetes, June 14, 1975.

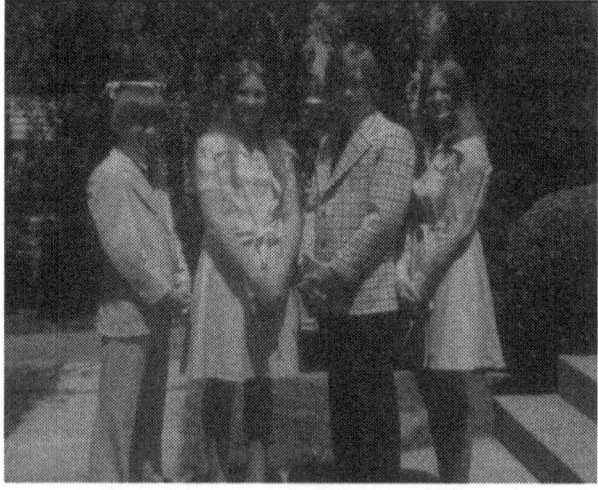

CHAPTER 2

DIABETES STRIKES AGAIN

Flu-Virus: Two years later in 1979, we had a new crisis to arise. While still trying to adapt to Doug becoming a diabetic, our oldest, David, then 21, and still living at home, began having frequent, severe headaches over a period of time.

December of that year had been a busy one for him. After working all day as a grocery clerk for Safeway, he spent a lot of his evenings shopping with Christmas coming on. He had been on the go, it seemed, the whole month of December. If he was not working, he was shopping – not getting much rest between times. Then just before the holiday, he came down with a bad flu-virus. At which time he became very sick. I took him to the emergency room, and there we were informed there was not much one could do for a virus, other than, giving something for fever and drinking lots of fluid. Although we had followed the doctor's orders, he still ran a high temperature between 102-103 for nearly two days straight.

He had been excited prior to that, as this was a "big" Christmas for him. He had bought Margie Bailey, his high school sweetheart an engagement ring, and his Dad and I a complete stereo-system with cabinet. Even though David was so sick Christmas morning, he smiled weakly as we each opened packages from him. Pleasing him that he had made our Christmas a happy one!

In Denial: Shortly after New Years Day, David came home from work not looking or feeling too well. As he came through the door that afternoon, he began telling me how thirsty he had been all day and how many times he had been to the bathroom. "At least a dozen times," he said. "I must be losing weight too, because my pants keep falling down," he continued, while showing me how many more notches he had put his belt buckle in.

Listening to him brought back ol' memories of his younger brother. Hearing the symptoms and seeing the weight loss were all signs I should have been aware of. This couldn't be, I thought. Not David too! I could not imagine David becoming a diabetic too. It was impossible! After all, we already had one son with diabetes. Thinking that it had to be something else, I told him that it was probably nothing to worry about other than just being overly tired, and worn down from just having had the flu. "If your symptoms don't subside, though," I said, "I'll get you a doctor's appointment."

Vic and I had plans that evening to go see his Aunt Maxine, who was visiting her sister, Hazel, Vic's mom. With her living in Roanoke, Virginia, we took every chance we could to see her when she came to visit. When asking David if he thought he would be all right while we were gone? "Sure!" he replied. "I'm going over to Margie's this evening anyway."

8

Our nice visit was short-lived, though. While there, I received a phone call from Doug telling me that he had given David one of his diastix strips to test his urine with. "It showed up dark brown," he announced, in an anxious tone. We both knew just what that meant - extremely high sugar passed through the urine. Doug was now trying to tell me something that I had tried to ignore earlier. There was a possibility that David was a diabetic too!

With teenagers coming and going, Doug was not around when David came home from work that afternoon. He had seen him only prior to his calling me. When asking him what made him think of checking David's urine? "He's got all the symptoms I had, mom," he answered, in a high pitch tone. "Don't you remember?" Having been in denial, I did not think once in having David check his urine that afternoon.

Through tear filled eyes as I told Vic, his mom, and his aunt, what Doug had just told me, their heads hung. Leaving his mom's shortly thereafter, we arrived home to find Margie had taken David to the Emergency Room. At the hospital that night, blood and urine tests were taken. With results revealing a 270 blood sugar reading, and a +4 sugar reading in the urine, they did nothing but send him back home. To this day, we have no logical reason to why this was done.

Doctor Kent on his rounds the next morning, had a hospital staff call us around 7:00 a.m., telling us that the doctor wanted David admitted. With further testing when he arrived, David was diagnosed as a Diabetic that day, on January 6, 1980. Just two years and four months after Doug was diagnosed.

God's Will: Vic and I were completely devastated by it all. After all, we did not have diabetes, and there again, knew of no one in the immediate family that did. So many unsolved questions went through our minds. The girls were fine. Why the boys? With them being the oldest and the youngest? It was all so hard to understand.

Dr. Greenhalgh, our family doctor taking the case, informed us that it was quite unusual for two siblings to inherit the disease. Especially, with neither parent a diabetic. The doctor said, David's probably stemmed from the past virus he had just had, and Doug's inherited because of the age he came down with it.

The doctor also told us that Vic and I could be carrying the gene; whereas, one or both of us could come down with diabetes ourselves later in life. "As late as your forties or fifties," he said. Diabetes at this age is called the maturity-onset, now called Type 2 or non-insulin-dependent. This form is not as severe as the Type 1 (insulin-dependent diabetes), which can be controlled by pill form.

I came to the conclusion that it was just God's will that both our boys were diabetic. Having found some relief and comfort thinking so. I thought with David a diabetic, God was showing Doug he was not alone – he would have David to lean on. He would share; they would share together this terrible disease that was inflicted upon them.

Doug had good and bad days dealing with his diabetes. Not just physically, but emotionally as well. Needing assurance to help him cope and withstand the everyday burden of being a diabetic, Doug prayed a lot through this difficult time. Telling me how much better he would feel by having done so.

David's Coping: David's hospital stay was five days. He was well controlled on just 12 units of NPH insulin in the hospital, but was discharged on 14. Having frequent insulin reactions at home, they tried him on the pill form instead. With persistent high blood sugar readings after that, it did not take long to find out which therapy would be best for him. Insulin injections would become a daily routine for him as well.

Unlike his brother, David had, and still has, a dislike for needles. When given directions on how to give injections, he was informed to watch for air-bubbles that may develop in the syringe, and what would happen if there was one. Finding that an air-bubble injected could be fatal, by stopping one's heart, freaked him out. Also the fact, that injecting into a vein can cause sudden insulin shock, an instant drop in blood sugar, did not help matters either. Which happened to him on two different occasions, which he says, "Isn't a pleasant experience."

Also unlike his brother, he had a hard time recognizing signs of high and low blood sugar when he was first diagnosed. Although he did well with his diet, he still fought a continuous battle with insulin reactions. His doctor referred to him as a "Brittle Diabetic" - word

11

used for tightly controlled. David becoming a diabetic seemed to bond he and Margie closer than ever. Planning to marry that coming June, they decided to do so earlier. With David diagnosed just three months prior, he and Margie made plans for a beautiful church wedding. They became husband and wife on April 5, 1980. Having bought a home, they settled in Stafford, about a 20-minute drive from Woodbridge.

Terrifying Ordeal: In the early part of October 1980, six months after David and Margie were married, we received a phone call early one Sunday morning. Vic had answered, and I could tell by the way he was talking that something bad had happened. "Margie's on the phone," Vic yelled out to me. Picking up the extension, I heard our "hysteric" daughter-in-law telling Vic about David. "He's in-coherent," she sobbed. "He fell out of bed and his whole body is jerking. He has like…foam coming from his mouth. I don't know what to do! I tried giving him some sugar, but he keeps knocking it out of my hand." "I called the rescue squad," she said, "but they haven't arrived yet. What should I do?" she asked frantically.

Listening to Margie, we could hear David in the background making all kinds of loud distressing sounds. We knew right away he was having a severe insulin reaction, and that time could mean a matter of "life or death." Having had a prescription for Glucagon, an injectable preparation for use in treating severe low blood sugar in case of an emergency such as this, we told Margie we would be right there.

While Vic went to get the truck, I ran and got the Glucagon and needle. By the time I got outside, Vic was already backing out of the driveway. Running, I grabbed the door and jumped in! As I prepared the needle, Vic broke every speed limit en route. We prayed for a policeman to stop us for speeding, with hopes he could lead us there even faster. That did not happen! "Where's a cop when ya' need 'em," we fumed. Though we had made the trip in record time, we were relieved to see the ambulance was already there.

Margie met us at the door, informing us that the ambulance had just arrived. "They couldn't find our house!" she cried, as tears ran down her mascara-streaked face. Entering their bedroom, we found David lying on the floor. In a semi-coma state, he was tossing his head from side to side. His eyes were wide open, but unseeing. He was not aware to what was going on. "Lord help us!" I thought, seeing the shape he was in.

The ambulance having no medical supplies for insulin shock, I immediately tried to administer the needle I had previously prepared. Finding this quite impossible with his moving about, Vic injected the needle. With it being done only by the aid of a sheriff's officer, whom at that time had a knee in David's chest and holding his arms down. Unaware what he was saying, he loudly repeating over and over, "I'm sick.... I'm sick".... as they wheeled him by stretcher to the ambulance.

Arriving at Potomac Hospital he was immediately connected to an IV, which led a steady stream of glucose into his bloodstream to help bring his blood sugar back to a normal range. Although he had been given the Glucagon shot Vic gave him, as well as the glucose by IV at the hospital, he still stayed unconscious for three long hours. Lifting his head at times, he stared blankly as he uttered how sick he was after having dry-heaved. Still repeating the same words – "I'm sick.... I'm sick".... over and over again.

All during this time, Margie, Vic, and I stayed vigil by his bedside. Holding his hand, talking to him, and silently praying. After what seemed an eternity, he became conscious. Lifting his head and looking around, he asked, bewildered, "Where am I?" Relieved, all I could say upon replying was: "Welcome back Son!"

Looking into his eyes then I could tell he was all right. With the glassy look gone, his eyes appeared bright and clear. David did not, and has not to this day, remembered anything about his near fatal death. After hearing about it all, he says, "I'm glad I didn't!" "I do remember Margie and I went to dinner the evening before, and then went walking through the shopping mall," he recalled.

Not being a diabetic for long, David did not realize how much sugar he was burning off by doing all the walking he had done that evening. Not having a blood monitor to check his blood sugar with, like Doug, he relied on the urine strips to get his blood sugar reading. Eating very little after arriving home that night, he went to bed thinking everything was all right. "I woke up a couple of times early that Sunday morning feeling real tired and weak," he remembered. "I tried getting up, but I didn't have the energy. That's all I know about it," he'd said.

We thank God to this very day that this happened on the weekend instead of a weekday. If Margie had been at work, we would no longer have him with us today!

Having a fear after this episode, David and Margie put their house up for sale to move closer to family in Woodbridge.

Wanting a Family: Anxious to start a family, they were somewhat hesitant. "I don't want my children having to endure all the problems that comes with Diabetes," David had said. "I know what it's like and what it can do to you!"

Confiding with their doctor, he assured them that having children with Diabetes was much greater if the mother was a diabetic, more so than the father being one. Upon heeding the advice, on March 1, 1982, their first born, Jennifer Evelyn arrived. Then, just two years and seven months later on October 7, 1984, their second daughter, Jessica Katherine was born. David and Margie could not have been happier! Their life was complete, two beautiful girls with good health, and no signs of diabetes.

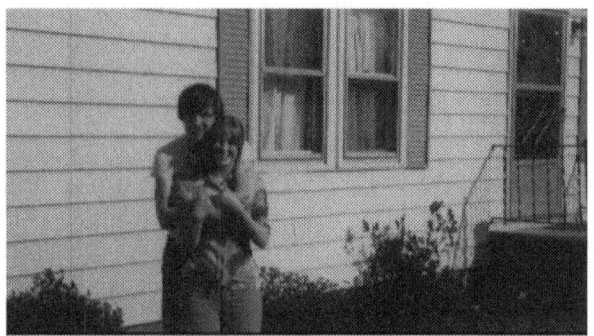

David and Margie in 1980 at their home in
Stafford shortly before he had his near fatal
episode with low blood sugar.

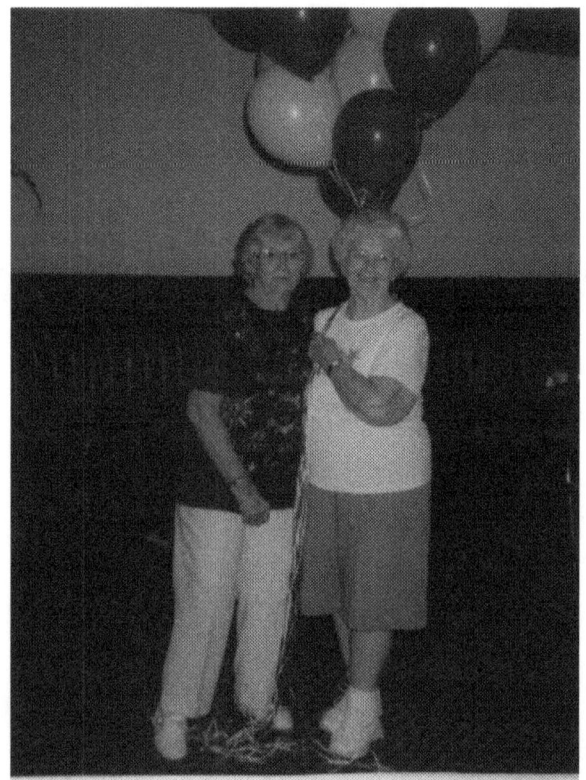

Virginia "Hazel" Tuck (Granny)
celebrates her 80th Birthday, posing with
her only sister, Maxine, July 20, 2001.

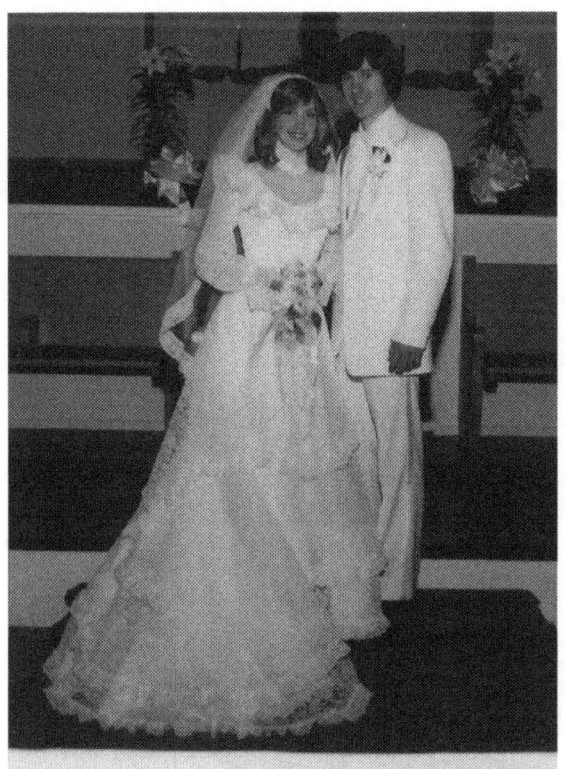

David and Margie's Wedding Day
April 5, 1980

CHAPTER 3

GOLDEN OPPORTUNITY * HYPERGLYCEMIA

In April of 1981, Doug married at age 18. Since they were both young and immature, the marriage ended in less than two years. Prior to his divorce, he had been involved in stock car racing with friend, Phil Poole. Doug was working for Potomac Steel Construction Company when he first met Phil. Having owned a race car, Phil would go to Potomac Steel to purchase supplies for his car. While there one day, Phil found out Doug's interest in stock cars. Having discovered they had both lived in the same sub-division, he asked Doug if he would be interested in helping him out with his race car. Doug did not think twice on taking him up on his offer. "Sure," he answered. "I'd love to help out!"

Diabetes pried on Doug's mind a lot, so getting involved in racing helped to keep his mind on something other than his medical condition constantly. Shortly afterward, Phil announced he would be going out of town for the weekend and would not be there to race. "If you want," he told Doug, "you can drive my race car while I'm gone." Doug was overwhelmed with excitement, as Phil had given him a golden opportunity to do something he had always wanted to do.

As Vic and I sat nervously in the stands that Saturday night watching him race for the very first time, we could not believe how well he was doing. Round and round he went, passing one car after another – going faster and faster. Then…. only after hitting the wall in turn four did we later learn, that the accelerator had stuck and that he had no brakes!

No wonder you were passing everyone out there, we later teased. Doug was devastated he had wrecked Phil's car. What would Phil say? he thought. "It wasn't my fault!" Doug told us. "After all, one can go through the turns just so fast." Upon seeing the car when Phil arrived home, he just chuckled. "No problem Doug," he told him, "We'll just fix her up and go again."

Race Fever: As crew chief, Doug had worked with Phil for four years. Out of the blue one day at the age of 22, Doug decided he wanted a race car of his own. Knowing Doug wanted to go on his own, Phil gave him an old car that he had bought for spare parts. With the 1972 Pontiac Catalina sitting in an abandoned field, it was towed home to become one of Doug's most gratifying and greatest challenges with stock car racing.

He could not wait to get started. So that fall in 1985, with very little money, he started repairing. First, by gutting it, a slang word used for stripping all the insides of the car out, including the windows. He then installed a roll-cage, racing instrument equipment, and a racing engine that he worked days modifying to his perfection. Last, but not least, he painted it bright red and placed a big white number 12 on the side of the door. Now that the car was ready there was only one thing lacking – sponsorship. Knowing just where to go, he made an appointment with our family doctor, John S. Greenhalgh. Knowing Doug and his love for racing, and out of the goodness of his heart, the doctor gave him sponsorship – putting Doug on cloud nine. He then appointed his Dad as crew chief, and with additional sponsor backing from family members, he was all set to go. We had never seen him so happy!

In spring of 86, his very first year racing as a rookie driver, Doug finished with a Championship. He continued his racing for the next seven years, competing in four different divisions. He had won back-to-back championships with 10 wins in each, and was voted "most Popular" team each year.

He was in the winner's circle 30 times during those seven years, with one of these memorable wins for the "Race For a Cure." Which was held at Old Dominion Speedway in Manassas, Virginia, to benefit the "Juvenile Diabetes Foundation". Diane Axline, who was head scorer for Old Dominion during that time, and to whom had two sons with Diabetes also, organized it. Our family teamed up with Diane, as well as other sponsors, drivers, and everyone in the stands that night to help make it a successful event.

Doug has received numerous plaques, trophies, and has had several newspaper articles written on him during his years of racing. Although past years were glorifying for him, it would change, though, in the following to come...

Hyperglycemia: On October 15, 1986, David had yet another battle with his diabetes. But this time, he had too much sugar in his blood instead of too little. Late that evening he began experiencing a variety of symptoms, such as, nausea, fatigue, loss of appetite, and deep rapid breathing, saying when he took a deep breath, he would get an awful smell. "Similar to bleach," he'd said. Causing him to have a burning sensation through his nose with every breath he took.

Calling the Emergency Room at Potomac Hospital about his symptoms, he was told that it was probably high blood sugar. They said he should do some sort of exercising to help bring it down. Feeling fatigued from high blood sugar, as well as having put in a day's work, and now being 11 p.m., David had said, "I certainly didn't feel like doing "jumping Jacks" as suggested!"

Not realizing what was happening to him for sure, he took it on his own and went to the hospital to be checked out. With test revealing a 600 blood sugar reading, he was admitted overnight. Knowing the erratic changes he had been having with blood sugar, the next morning one of the nurses told David that it would be wise to invest in a blood monitor. With his insurance now covering some of the cost, he took her advice. His diabetes has been more accurate and easier to control since then.

The following two years things went smoothly for David and Doug in spite of their Diabetes. David's blood sugar stabilized since he had the blood monitor, and though Doug did not have one, he seemed to be

doing fine. All was going well.

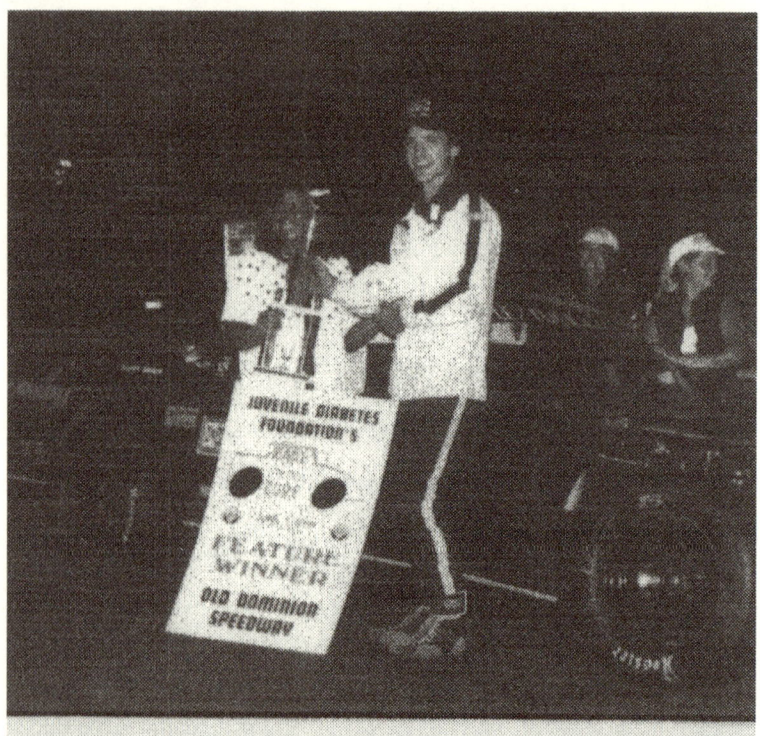

Diane Axline, Chairwoman of the "Race for
The Cure", presents a trophy to Doug Tuck,
winner of the 25-lap Grand Stock event,
June 1, 1990.

CHAPTER 4

NEW HORIZONS

In July 1988, Doug was in his third year of racing. With seven wins in mid-season, he was looking toward a third straight championship. His luck ended, though, due to a blown engine and mechanical problems that plagued him. With lack of financial backing, he had to sell his race car.

Meantime, car owners, Carl Doyle and wife Shelly, were looking for a driver for their race car. A close friend of ours told the Doyles that Doug would make them a good driver, now that he sold his race car. Knowing his track record, the Doyles approached Doug to team up with them for the next year. In the spring of 1989, the Doyle/Tuck Racing Team made their first debut together.

In late fall, on November 2, 1989, Doug married for the second time. This marriage, like the first, lasted a short time – just 16 months. Short relationships prior to, and a lack of communication, played a big role in their failed marriage.

Race For A Cure: From 1989 to 1991, Doug was still driving for the Doyles. A team for three years, they never won a race until Saturday, June 1, 1991, when he won the "Race for a Cure" at ODS, his home track. Doug started the Motor Grand Stock 25-lap feature on the outside pole in their number 11 Chevrolet Monte Carlo, leading the entire distance to pick up the win.

A diabetic himself, he could not have won on a better night. He was a very happy driver in victory lane, and will certainly remember this race as a memorable one, as well as family and crewmembers! Also during this time, Doug became good friends with Sharon Marlin, a friend of the Doyle's – who would later become his third wife.

Modified: In the spring of 1992, Doug began his seventh year of competitive racing. During that time there was a new class forming called the Modified – open wheel cars with speeds faster than the previous ones he had driven. The Doyles invested in one of these and Doug was excited. He had always wanted to drive a late model, (highest class up in stock-car-racing) and thought this would be the closest thing to it.

All modifieds run 8-cylinder motors, but the Doyles on a fixed racing income took their 6-cylinder out of the grand-stock and put it in the modified. Knowing a lot about 6-cylinder motors, Carl had no problem getting it to run as fast as the 8-cylinders. And that he did! It not only ran well, but also had its own unique sound. One did not have to see, nor know when Doug was on the track. You could tell just by the sound of the motor as he went by!

On Thursday evening, March 12, 1992, Doug and Carl had been working on the modified at a garage several miles from home. While driving home later that night, Doug was thinking of all the things he had yet to do before race season started, when suddenly, his right eye became blurred. By the time he arrived home, he could barely see out of it. Alarmed, he called his Optometrist the next morning and made an appointment to see him that day. Finding a massive hemorrhage behind Doug's right eye, Dr. Grober referred him to an Ophthalmologist Specialist. Which he told him, "Go see him right away!"

Diabetic Retinopathy: Five days later on March 17, Doug had his first consultation with Dr. John Baldinger - a skilled Ophthalmologist, whom was located in Fairfax, VA. Diagnosed with **Proliferative Diabetic Retinopathy** that day, we were told if left untreated, it could lead to permanent vision loss. Being a diabetic for 15 years, and progressed to this stage, Dr. Baldinger told Doug diabetes caused it.

Although Diabetic Retinopathy is considered one disease, there are many different types. Doctors have classified different kinds of Retinopathy to help them understand how one's vision is being affected. Two main categories are **Nonproliferative Retinopathy** (when blood vessels leak, then close) and **Proliferative Retinopathy** (when new blood vessels grow, or proliferate).

Progressing to the "proliferative" stage, as was Doug's case, due to inadequate blood flow, the retina begins to generate new blood vessels to replace the vessels that have closed up. When these new vessels form, they are abnormal, fragile, and grow inappropriately. This causes blood to leak inside the eye, which is why Doug had clouded, blurry vision. If untreated, the new vessels may even cause the retinal cells to detach from the back of the eye, resulting in severe visual loss or blindness.

Dr. Baldinger told Doug that he would have to use laser on his eye. "We'll wait a couple of days, though," he said. "To see if the blood clears any on its own. The damage has already been done," he informed us. With him saying that his eye would be all right other than not seeing too well."

Having made an appointment, Doug returned two days later on March 19, the day before his 29th birthday. With three different laser patterns used for whatever one's problem may be, Doug was told he would be given panretinal treatment. Saying the laser would be applied around the fovea to reduce new blood vessel growth. Given the option of anesthetic for numbness to his eye prior to treatment, Doug chose tropical drops instead of the needle.

Watching as Dr. Baldinger began, I could see Doug's legs grasp the laser machine stand. With each sap of the laser beam, his legs grasped tighter and tighter. Although Doug was given drops of anesthetic to prevent discomfort, after 30 some saps it became very painful for him. Knowing the pain he had went through, the doctor praised him afterward saying how well he had done.

Southside Speedway: With his eye doing better after three-laser treatments, in two weeks time, Doug was back racing. He did well with his 6-cylinder, and was soon well known within the division. Most of his fellow-drivers could not believe he was driving a modified with a

6-cylinder motor. They were also bound and determined not to let his 6-cylinder beat their eight!

The first race of the season was in April of 1992. It was held at Southside Speedway in Richmond, Virginia, where Doug started pole-position that night in a 50-lap feature. When the green flag dropped, he took the lead and held it until a caution came out on lap 39. With Doug in the lead on the re-start, he was hit and spun out by a driver, who pushed his car too hard trying to get around him. Although it was not Doug's fault, he had to re-start in the back to end up finishing fifth in the race. He did not win that night, but his 6-cylinder race car was recognized as one to beat!

Physical: Prior to his eye problem, Doug was not under the care of a Diabetic Specialist. He had been getting his physicals at a local health clinic by a doctor that was highly recommended. Having a physical in early February 1992, the doctor informed Doug that his blood work showed some irregularities. With counts slightly higher on his Glucose (sugar) and his Creatinine count (kidney), and lower counts on three different elements with one of them indicating he was anemic, he was told he had to have a series of Vitamin B shots. After beginning his series of Vitamin B shots, he said in time, he did not feel any different than before.

The doctor, concerned about Doug's blood results with him just turning 29, told him, "If you want any children, you should have them before age 32. Or no later than 35," he stressed. Doug was upset about his blood results, as well as the thought of never having children, which he had looked forward to one day.

Moving In Together: Spring and summer came and went, and with racing over for the year he had other important plans to attend to. In the fall of November 1992, he and his girlfriend, Sharon, rented an apartment and moved in together with no future plans of marriage. Paranoid from past failed marriages, Doug thought their relationship would be better if they just lived together. Sharon liked the arrangement as well, and their lives seemed uncomplicated. Sharon held a high position job with TRW with an above average income, and Doug was working for General Heating & Air Conditioning Company with good hours and pay. The only downfall they had to contend and worry about was Doug's eyes.

Keeping a close watch, the following month in late December, Dr. Baldinger found deterioration in Doug's left eye. Whereupon, one week before Christmas, he had his first laser treatment – not being quite as bad as the right one.

Surprise Announcement: In early January 1993, we received news that Sharon was pregnant. "The due date is August 26," they exclaimed, all excited with both wanting a child. Doug was looking forward to having a boy. Due to the Tuck's generation slowly diminishing, he was hoping for a son to carry on the name.

When Sharon had a sonogram, they were told they would be having a girl. Doug was a little disappointed at first when finding out. He said, "If I had a son, I could take him huntin' and fishin', and he could tell all the kids at school his daddy was a race car driver! I could even teach him how to drive a race car!" "You can do all those things with a girl too!" we told him laughing. "Having a girl, I'll just spoil her and be over protective," he replied right back. "Not only that," he said, "when she gets married, she'll no longer carry my name! "Just wait until she gets here," we told him. "You'll think otherwise."

Setback: Although Doug's eyes improved some it did not last for long. With him already having had three laser treatments to his right eye just a year prior, on May 4, he had to have additional laser. Then, just twenty-one days later on May 25, he had to have repeated laser treatment to his left eye, which he had first five months prior. Things did not let up for him. With blood vessels rupturing in his left eye less than a month later, on June 16, he had to have repeated laser on that one again. Doug was devastated by it all. His eyesight was a major concern for him as it would be for anyone. But there was one thing he was not going to give up if he could help it, and that was his racing. It seemed, that was the only thing that kept him going.

In the beginning, he did not want the Doyles to know he had an eye problem, for fear they would not let him drive for them. "If Curtis can do it, I can too," he remarked bravely, speaking of Curtis Markham. Who at that time was a late-model stock car driver - being one of

Old Dominion Speedway's best. Curtis had lost an eye when he was younger, which did not hinder him in any way – especially in a race car. He later went on to become a Busch car driver in NASCAR.

Limited Schedule: Doug's racing was limited, driving a modified for the (ARA) American Racing Association, due to a touring schedule that involved seven different tracks throughout Virginia. Because of the time and expense associated with touring, the Doyles decided they would race locally at their home track as scheduled. Doing very little traveling to other tracks did not upset Doug any. In fact, it pleased him. Not because of his wanting to race, but due to the lateness that would be involved traveling the distance. He never was a night owl as one might call it. Even as a kid, he was the only one out of our four that was the first to bed at night and the first to rise in the morning.

Although Doug came close to winning a regular feature race with the modified, he never did. However, he did win two (5) lap trophy dashes. The trophy dash was run prior to the main event, with the top four qualifiers being inverted for the race. Doug won both of these at his home track, where he received large ARA plaques for his achievement. No one knew, or would have known about his poor eyesight at the time, for his driving performance was nothing but superb.

New Arrival: Finding a house during this time, Doug and Sharon moved from their apartment on the other side of town in August 1993, to a home they had found in our sub-division. It was a rental home, to which they put a two-year-lease on. Later that month on the 27th, just one day late from her due date, Sharon gave birth to Melissa Anne at Fairfax Hospital.

Doug could not have been happier! "She looks just like me!" doesn't she?" he would ask beaming, as friends and family members came to see their new arrival. He was so proud! Melissa looked a lot like her daddy when first born, and more so as she has gotten older, as well as having a lot of her daddy's ways.

Since then, he has spoiled her to a certain extent, but above all, has taught her respect and discipline. As time goes on, Doug will have taken her fishin', go-cart racing, and when asked who's the best race car driver, she'll answer, "My daddy is!"

Doug is over-protective with Melissa. She is his life, the child he has wanted for so long. He no longer thinks of his name being carried on.

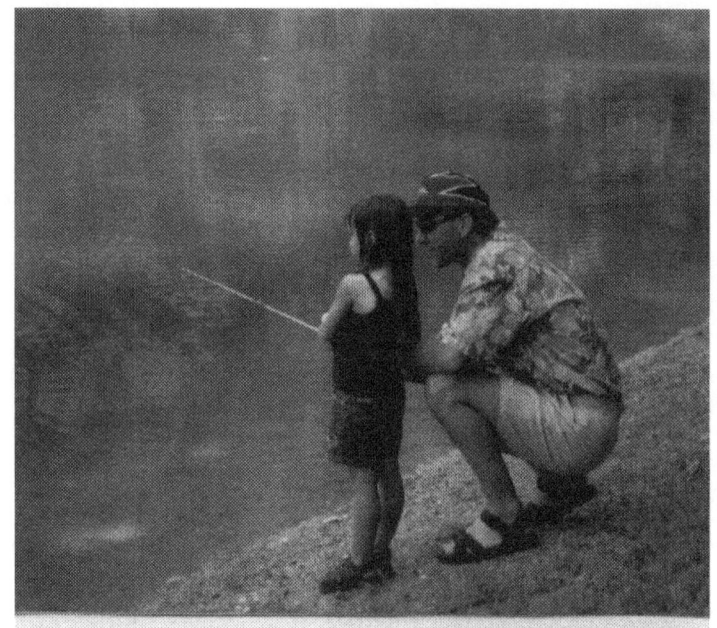

Doug teaching Melissa how to fish in the pond at
Issiac Walton, where he and Sharon were married.

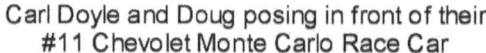

Carl Doyle and Doug posing in front of their
#11 Chevolet Monte Carlo Race Car

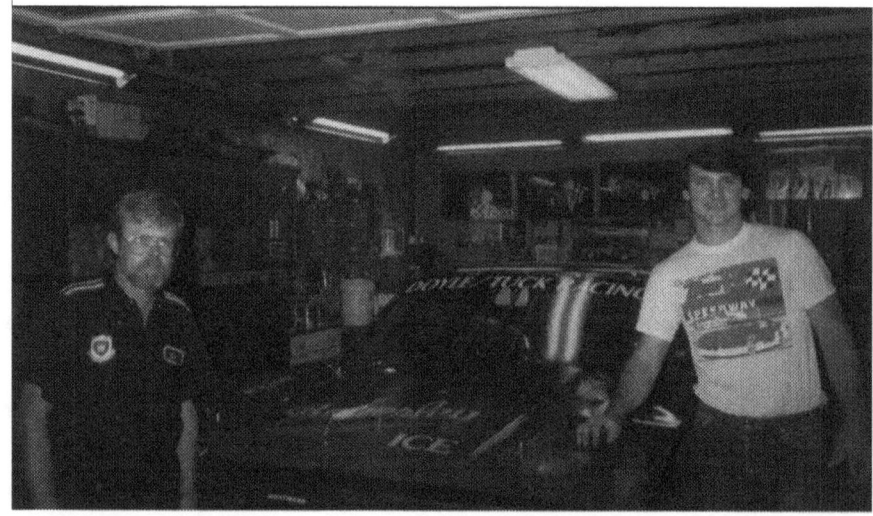

Modified Trophy Dash Win at Old Dominion Speedway.

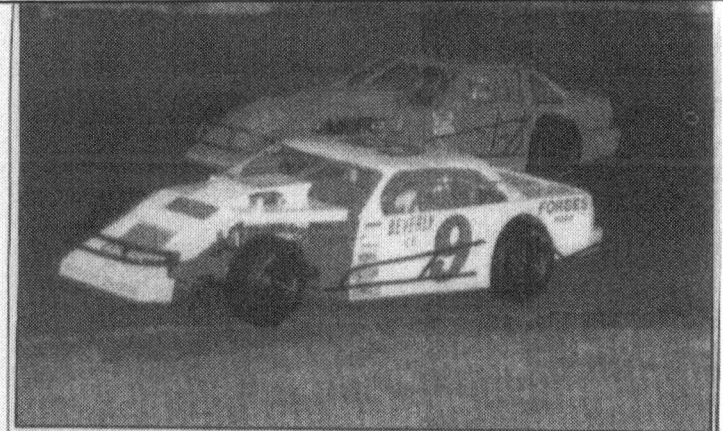

Former Motorworld Grand Stock campaigner Doug Tuck (9) won the special dash event over Johnny Minor (15), who came home a close second...

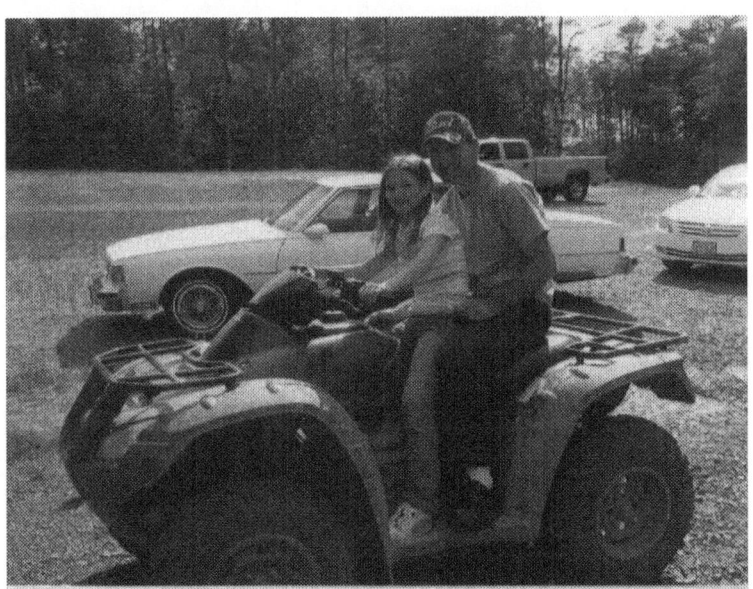

Melissa 11, takes her dad (Doug), for a ride on a four wheeler at her Aunt Laura and Uncle Alex's, May 21, 2005

CHAPTER 5

DOCTOR'S CONCERN

In late summer of 1993, Doug's work was no longer a chore, it became a burden to him. Working for a Heating and Refrigeration Co., his job was installing heat pumps and running electrical cable. With a job that required heavy lifting, as well as good eye contact, Doug was having a difficult time. Not wanting any pressure put on Doug's eyes, Dr. Baldinger told him, "You can work, but don't do any heavy lifting." Although he continued working, it was not easy. He did not do any lifting, but had a difficult time seeing close up work that had to be done.

By November, Doug's right eye continued to get worse. Having trouble seeing, he made an appointment with Dr. Baldinger. Seeing blood in the vitreous (a transparent gel-like substance that fills the chamber behind the lens of the eye) the doctor told Doug he would have to do a (vitrectomy). A medical term used to remove the vitreous, which is usually performed only after all other treatments have been attempted.

"Laser will be of no help to you now," the doctor advised. Telling him that the bleeding was caused by the vitreous pulling on the new 'weak' blood vessels.

With the doctor being concerned about a retinal detachment, due to the vitreous pulling on the retina, he wanted to correct the problem before it happened. Dr. Baldinger informed us as well, that the vitreous (the gel-transparent substance) found in diabetics felt sticky compared to non-diabetics. He gave us no explanation to why that is, other than saying he had found the condition in other diabetics. With him explaining, that the sticky substance pulls on the new blood vessels, and makes them bleed.

We were concerned at that time as well, about Doug's blood pressure. He had mentioned several times about feeling a throbbing behind his eyes. "Like a heart beat feels," he would say. We mentioned this to Dr. Baldinger, which he replied that high blood pressure could have contributed to Doug's eye problem. When asking if he had a recent checkup, Doug told him about the recent physicals he had, where no blood pressure was taken at such time. Having to be evaluated prior to surgery, as well as under the care of a diabetic doctor, the doctor referred him to Dr. Michael F. Ball, an Endocrinologist. "Go see him," he said. "He'll be able to detect if anything is wrong."

Dr. Ball's Visit: Doug's visit with Dr. Ball took place on November 3, 1993. At which time he was diagnosed with high blood pressure, and a creatinine count of 2.9 with a normal reference range 0.5-1.3. We were also informed his glycated hemoglobin count (useful for assessing long-term glucose in diabetes) was a 14, with poor control associated with a count of 12 or more.

I went with Doug that day to Dr. Ball's as I have with all other doctor appointments in the past. When Doug's name was called, Dr. Ball greeted us outside his door.

Introducing himself, he told us to take a seat. Whereupon, this tall, highly educated man who takes his profession seriously, came down hard on Doug. Having lab report before him and Doug's history with diabetes and recent eye problem, Dr. Ball began to lecture. He began asking question, and he wanted answers. Not any of this, "I don't know," or "I can't remember" stuff! Dr. Ball was loud and harsh sounding at times. Giving, what seemed, a lengthy scolding. At one point it got so bad, I thought Doug might get up and walk out!

Looking stern at Doug, he told him, "You are 30-years-old Doug. It's up to you if you want to live a long, or short life." Having followed by telling him, he would have to take two-insulin shots a day instead of just one. "To get you in control," he said firmly. Dr. Ball then told him how to re-adjust his insulin with his diet and activities. Informing him as well, that his high blood pressure most likely contributed to his eye problem.

To keep check on his kidney function, he referred him to Robert E. Greenspan a Nephrologist, located in Woodbridge, not far from home. Giving Doug a prescription for his blood pressure, Dr. Ball remarked, "Come back to see me in three months!"

Doug was not in the best of mood when leaving. He not only had to worry about his eyes now, but also his blood pressure, his creatinine count, as well as his diabetes out of control. Plus, given a doctors lecture on top of it all, just left him feeling uneasy and agitated that day. "Ya' know mom," he said, on the way out, "I got so mad in there, I almost walked out! Then I realized, he was saying all that for my sake. Guess... he thought I wasn't takin' good enough care of myself." "I thought I was," he said, looking down.

Silent Killer: Although Doug's diabetes was not controlled during that time, he did not feel all that bad. He just was not aware of how serious his condition had gotten. And with him muscular and very healthy looking at 6-foot-2 and weighing 197 lbs, one would never guess he had diabetes and all the complications that he had endured.

Shortly after Dr. Ball's visit, our local TV-News-Channel, NBC, had a report one evening on hypertension, informing what all it could do to ones health if not treated. Untreated hypertension could cause damage to various organs and bodily systems that could lead to strokes, heart attacks, eye damage, kidney failure, and permanent damage to the vascular system. It also stated, that hypertension is often called the "Silent Killer" because symptoms are often lacking, and that the only way to know for sure if you have a problem is to have your blood pressure checked on a regular basis.

After hearing this, Doug and I reminisced about the doctor he had in the past. The one that had given him, what was suppose to be, good physicals. Doug had been under this doctor's care for nearly two years. Having had physicals and blood work on four different occasions. The doctor had to be aware during this time of Doug's poor health condition, as he had informed him of his creatinine count being elevated, as well as being anemic. In knowing all this, not once, did the doctor think of checking Doug's blood pressure!

"Are you sure he never checked your blood pressure?" I had asked Doug. "Blood pressure checks are always given when you have physicals." "I know what's done when you have your blood pressure checked," Doug snapped back. "I'm telling you, he never took it!"

Part of the physical routine, the doctor had given Doug an Electrocardiogram during one of his visits. Reading the results to Doug, that he had compared with David, whom he had previously given one, the doctor told him, "You have good heart! Much better than brothers." "You have good strong heart!" he repeated, by letting Doug know everything was all right.

"Now I know why the doctor said you have good strong heart," Doug snarled, in going back over this. "My dang blood pressure was sky high." With him thinking, that was causing his heart to beat so strong. "You should have seen the peaks on my electrocardiogram! They were twice as high as David's." If his blood pressure had been detected earlier and treated, we thought, it would have saved damage to his eyes and kidneys. Unfortunately, there is no turning back!

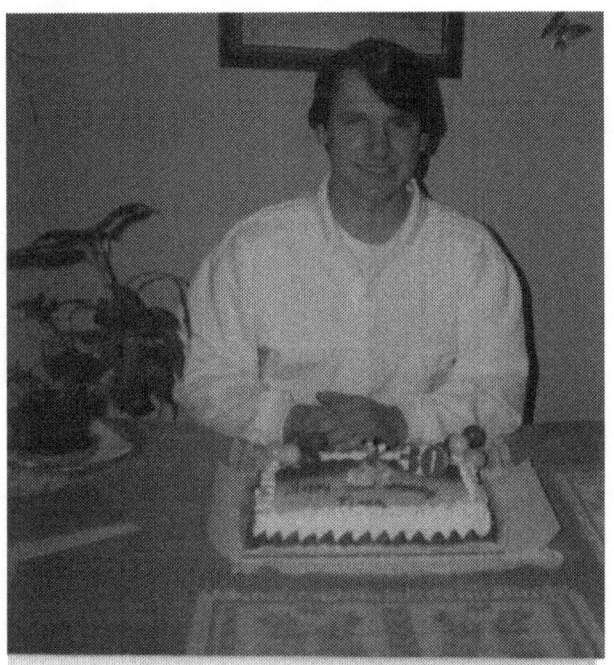

Doug's 30th Birthday, March 20, 1993 at the time he began lazer treatments on his eyes.

CHAPTER 6

EYE SURGERIES * DISABILITY

1ST **Major Eye Surgery:** On November 12, 1993, nine days after Dr. Ball's visit, Doug underwent his first major surgery on his right eye at Fairfax Hospital. During surgery, Dr. Baldinger would remove the vitreous and any remaining scar tissue pulling on the retina, caused from past laser treatment. The vitreous would be replaced with an air-bubble to help keep the retina in place. The doctor informed Doug prior to surgery that a repeat may be necessary if bleeding, or if a retinal detachment would occur anytime after.

Admitted as an outpatient, Doug was told he could stay overnight, or go home after surgery, if he felt up to it. The surgery went well, with not much discomfort other than a bad headache and some eye pain. He was sent home that evening with a prescription for pain and medicated eye drops. Doug was told to return the next morning to Dr. Baldinger's office to have his eye checked and rebandaged. Whereupon, he was told he would have to wear a patch over his eye for several days. After it was removed, he could barely see. Although alarmed, he was told prior, that it would be normal to expect temporary vision loss for a few days.

In having to insert a vitrectomy instrument and a light source probe through Doug's eye, it appeared red, inflamed and irritated – looking

40

as if he had a massive eye hemorrhage. The doctor assured Doug that the outer eye would clear in time, as the doctor's main concern was the clearing of blood from behind it. "Usually the blood clears up on its own," Dr. Baldinger told him, "which takes four weeks or so. If it doesn't, I'll have to go back in and do what they call a wash-out - syringe the blood out." We were told in not doing so would cause prolonged eyesight loss. Seven weeks later on December 30, he had additional laser applied to his left eye, with the blood still not cleared in his right one.

2ᴺᴰ Eye Surgery: Entering the New Year, things did not get any better. Less than two weeks later on January 11, 1994, Doug had to have repeated surgery on his right eye. With the blood still not clearing from past surgery, plus another hemorrhage, he underwent his first "washout" and additional laser. He wanted to come home again as an outpatient, but more pain and anesthesia than before prevented him from doing so.

I felt such sorrow as I stood by his bedside that evening, thinking how much he had been through thus far. Still very groggy from the anesthesia, he turned to Sharon and said, "Where's ... mom?" "Right behind you," she answered. "I'm right here," I told him, placing my hand on his shoulder. "How are you feeling? Are you in much pain?" Without answering, he turned and reached for my hand. Then squeezing lightly, he softly muttered three little words, "I wanna race."

Having the fear of losing his eyesight and never being able to race again was more than Doug could withstand. He loved racing. And unlike Diabetes with all its complications, racing was something he would have full control of. I tried to ensure him things would get better as he slowly drifted back to sleep.

Jobless: By spring of 1994, Doug was not doing well at all. After having right eye surgery just two months prior, he was back in Dr. Baldinger's office on March 11, for his fifth laser treatment on his left eye. During this period of his life, he could no longer see enough to drive, or even walk. Doug had to hold Sharon's arm to be led. During this difficult time, Sharon did all the financial supporting with him unable to work.

Knowing the financial struggle they were going through, I called our local Social Security office and the Juvenile Diabetes Foundation to see what they could do. Whereas, I was told by Social Security if he was not completely disabled, even if he had a child, there was nothing they could do. If you were a woman with a child you could get help, but if you were a man, well... that was entirely different.

The Juvenile Diabetes Foundation did offer to help pay for his insulin and needles, but as for any financial help – they did not do that either. Doug did have one good thing going for him. Unable to work for a long period of time, his job was good enough to let him continue paying on his premiums so he could keep his health insurance until he went back. With Doug's enormous doctor bills, this was a blessing for them.

3ᴿᴰ Eye Surgery: Although Doug had already had one washout on his right eye three and-a-half months prior, he was admitted to repeat the same procedure on April 28, 1994. Things just would not let up for him. It seemed he would no sooner get over one surgery, that he would be right back having another. Such was the case this time. Just six-and-a-half weeks later on June 14, Dr. Baldinger had to perform a vitrectomy on Doug's left eye, due to the same problem he had with the right one – the vitreous pulling on the new weak blood vessels, causing them to bleed.

From March '92 through June '94, Doug underwent five laser treatments, a vitrectomy, and two washouts on his right eye. As well as five laser treatments and a vitrectomy on his left one. Although, no washouts were done on the left eye, it still took several weeks for it to clear well enough to see.

Between all the laser treatments, major eye surgeries, and vision loss, he also had to contend with the worry of his blood pressure, kidneys, being jobless, his finances, and could no longer do what he loved - race. At this particular time, Doug at 31-years-old and at wits' end, felt his life crumbling beneath him. Although he had a lot to be thankful for, his coping was difficult during this period.

Medical Expense: Excluding hospital bills, the total cost for those two years of office visits, laser treatments, surgeries, scans, and ultrasounds performed on his eyes by Dr. Baldinger, totaled over $21,000.00.

The cost of Doug's medical bill was relatively small compared to what it could have been. Doug was greatful to Dr. Baldinger, for giving him discount rates because he was jobless at that time, and for health insurance as they paid a great amount.

"If it had all cost $100,000.00 it would have been worth it!" Doug exclaimed, happily, as he praised and credited Dr. Baldinger for restoring his eyesight. What a blessing we had for medical technology with him now having 20/20 vision.

Disability: Around the time of Doug's eye surgery in June 1994, Sharon was enduring burden of 'all' responsibilities. Overwhelmed by it all and wanting to know if Doug could get disability, she took it upon herself and recalled Social Security. Explaining his medical condition, she was told to make an appointment to present his case.

Sharon made an appointment for June 17, and I drove him to our local Social Security Administration Building in Manassas. He walked in with a patch on his eye from just having had surgery three days prior.

Giving Doug's medical history and the amount of time he was jobless, the clerical worker seemed very optimistic to his getting disability. "But first," she said, "You'll have to get an eye exam. To prove that your eyes are bad enough to qualify for benefits." Taking two months to get an appointment for his eye exam, it was performed on August 19, by a doctor who works through Social Services.

Doug was run through a series of test, which he thought he did not pass. The doctor did not tell him how the tests went that day, only to receive a letter two-and-a-half weeks later saying that his case had been denied. We could not believe it! If he was not satisfied and thought the decision was unjust, they informed that he could appeal it and reclaim in three months.

Doug's eyesight at the time the tests were done was very bad. And Doug feeling betrayed, did not think twice about appealing his case and reclaiming. Since he had to wait a certain amount of time before he was eligible to do so, he went to Dr. Baldinger telling him about his case being denied. "Dr. Baldinger, you know the condition of my eyes," Doug told him. "Inside and out. You know what I'm seeing! Can you write a letter to Social Security, so they'll know how bad my eyes are?" "Sure. I'll be glad too," the doctor replied, with it hard to believe the claim was rejected. At the proper time the reclaim was sent back in, as well as Dr. Baldinger sending his letter, stating, Doug's eye condition, and his opinion of Doug's working ability.

Creatinine Count Elevated: Also during this period, Doug made an appointment with a Nephrologist, a Kidney Specialist, to which he saw Dr. Greenspan on October 5, 1994. At such time he was diagnosed with a creatinine count of 4.4, whereas, just eleven months prior his count was 2.9 at Dr. Ball's office. Seeing his count elevated, Dr. Greenspan wanted to see him on a monthly basis.

Wanting to know more about Creatinine and its count with kidney function, I found: It is a byproduct of the normal growth and repair of muscle tissue, to which it's waste products are removed from the blood by the kidneys. By blood test, it's level or count is referred to as a number that is watched closely, and serves as an indicator of kidney function.

Although the early years of diabetes can show supernormal renal function, after ten years or more of diabetes, kidney function may begin to go downhill because of the microscopic scarring of capillaries and the small arteries in the kidney's filter system. Obtaining this knowledge, I realized then, that Doug's eye problem was related to the same circumstances as his kidneys were.

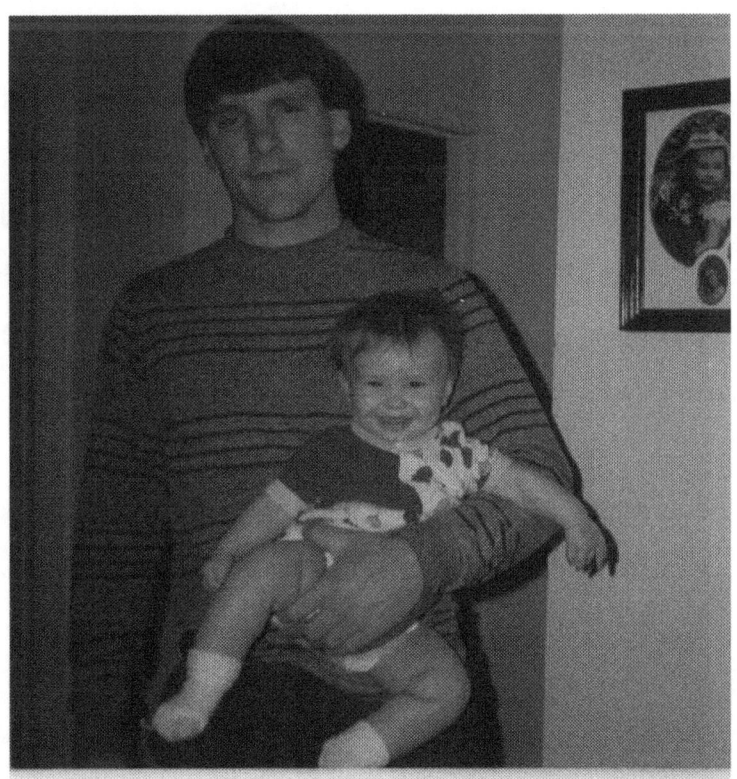

A sad looking Doug holds 9-month old Melissa
shortly after his second eye surgery, January 11, 1994

CHAPTER 7

GOOD AND BAD TIMES

Unable to work for over a year, and less than a month after Dr.Greenspan's visit, Doug was terminated from his job on October 28, 1994. And if that was not bad enough, three weeks later on November 17, he received another letter from Social Security saying his claim had been denied again! Then making matters worse, about a month-and-a-half later on December 28, his creatinine had gone up to 5.2, indicating that his kidney function was deteriorating more rapidly now.

Whereupon, Dr. Greenspan told Doug to cut down on the amount of protein he ate. Telling us that cutting down the amount of protein eaten is suspected of being another way to slow the process of kidney disease. In doing so, he wanted Doug to make an appointment with the dietitian. Little did we know then, that Doug was beyond help and in such a short time how things would change so drastically.

Attorney: Although we had worried about Doug's creatinine count going up, we were very thankful that his eyes were doing much better. Now being able to drive, he was helping his Uncle Alan and Aunt Carole in their coffee business. They could use his help and he could use the extra money.

Though still upset over the fact that he did not qualify for disability for the year he was not able to work, and feeling they owed him the money, he and Sharon decided to take action. Given a free initial consultation, they went to see an attorney that handles Social Security Disability cases on January 19, 1995.

There they learned one has to be totally blind before disability is approved. Having explained to the attorney at the time Doug took his test, that he was unable to see well enough to perform his job as well as drive his car, the attorney took this into consideration and refilled his disability claim. Stating, that it may be weeks before Doug would hear anything!

During this time, Doug had additional issues to deal with. Still helping his Uncle Alan, whom was a small businessman, there was no set-up for employment benefits. In bad need for health insurance after losing his when he was terminated, he knew it would cost him a fortune to get one on his own with his medical history. That is, if he could get one at all!

Racing Fever: By spring of 1995, Doug was still showing a slight increase in his creatinine each month in spite of watching his protein intake. With his eyes doing better and racing season coming up, he had just one thing on his mind at that time. He wanted to race.

Carl had put his modified up for sale the year before, when Doug was unable to drive for him. And with it not selling, he gave Doug the opportunity to buy it by giving him a good deal. He was anxious to be on his own again. He also thought he had something to prove, as he did not want anyone thinking he was handicapped in any way. He wanted to prove he could still do it! Sharon, Vic and I thought it was a good idea, knowing that the race car would occupy and help keep his spirits up. During this time he had all kinds of things going for him – the race car and getting married!

Wedding: Doug and Sharon had put off getting married for some time. Now, that he had no health insurance, they were thinking otherwise. Getting married would benefit them at this particular time, with Doug being covered through Sharon's insurance at work. Not only that, with Melissa going on two-years-old, they knew they owed her that. And the fact that they lived together for four years – why not get married! After all, they loved one another. The next couple of months were busy ones for them. They not only had a wedding to plan, they also had to find a new home with their two year-lease up on their rental one.

Doug and Sharon were married on a bright, sunny day on Saturday, May 6, 1995. The wedding was held at a lodge - overlooking a pond with numerous family and friends attending. It was a lovely wedding, with a beautiful bride, a handsome groom, and with Melissa as their pretty flower girl – a happy day where all seemed right. That bubble would burst, though, just eighteen days later. Taking us all into a turbulent turmoil, that would change our lives forever.

Devastating News: On May 24, eighteen days after their wedding, Doug went back to Dr. Greenspan for his monthly check-up. Diagnosed with a 10.1 creatinine count, the doctor informed us that Doug had lost 85 percent of his kidney function. "Have you been feeling any nausea?" he asked Doug. "No," he answered.

Looking concerned, the doctor told him, "When your creatinine reaches a 12, you'll have to go on dialysis. You will need to have a fistula placed in your arm as soon as possible," he told him. "It takes seven to ten days for the incision to heal after surgery, and four to six weeks for the fistula to fully develop enough for the dialysis needles. Hopefully, the fistula will be ready by the time you need it," he said.

Doug and I were completely stunned by Doctor Greenspan's diagnosis that afternoon, as three of the most dreadful, devastating and frightening words any patient and family member could hear from his or her physician are "you need dialysis."

Kidney Failure: Learning about kidney failure, we found there are two types: Acute and Chronic. Acute means the kidneys have suddenly, and usually temporarily, stopped working. This type of failure can often be reversed. Serious infections, severe diarrhea or vomiting, drug poisoning, surgery, injury or blockage of the kidneys may also cause acute kidney failure. When the source of the problem is treated, the kidneys usually begin to function properly again.

Chronic kidney failure is a permanent condition. Once it occurs, the kidneys will not regain their function. Chronic kidney failure may be caused by hereditary conditions or diseases, or may be caused by ongoing medical conditions like hypertension or diabetes. Chronic kidney disease will eventually lead to scarring of the kidneys and "End Stage Renal Disease" (ESRD).

Diagnosed with (ESRD) means that the kidneys can no longer function to remove wastes and fluids from the bloodstream. A person with this will need to rely on medical treatment to replace the lost kidney function. There are several types of treatment for kidney failure. The two main treatments are Dialysis and Transplantation. Each patient and his/her doctor must decide on the form of treatment, which is best for that person.

Normally, ESRD patients produce little or no urine at all, prior to going on Dialysis. This was not Doug's case. His urinating stayed normal until he started Dialysis, whereupon, his urine was not as great as it was prior too.

No one would ever guess that Doug's creatinine had reached a 10. He was not sick, nor did he look sick. This all happened so fast. Too fast – just like his eyes did. The doctor could not tell us why such things happen this way, only that it can, and does happen.

With Doug having a 10.1 creatinine count, Dr. Greenspan did not waste anytime that day by referring him to Mauricio D. Bas, Jr., a Thoracic & Vascular Surgeon, whom was located directly across the street from his office. "Go make an appointment now!" the doctor ordered. Being an emergency case, we got in to see Dr. Bas that day. To which the doctor explained, in complete detail, the surgery procedure that Doug would soon be going through.

Dr. Bas told us that a person's bloodstream is connected to the artificial kidney through a Fistula or Graft. Telling us that a fistula is a surgical connection between an artery and a vein. Saying it is usually done in the arm, but sometimes in the leg. We were also informed when making a graft, an artificial blood vessel is used to connect an artery and a vein.

Fistula Surgery: On May 25, the day after seeing Dr. Bas, Doug was admitted to Potomac Hospital. During surgery, the doctor would create a fistula instead of a graft, due to Dr. Greenspan's preference.

Dr. Bas would make an access (opening into) the blood vessels, above Doug's wrist on left forearm. With the blood vessels exposed, Dr. Bas made a surgical connection between Doug's artery and vein. As the blood flows through this new connection it causes the vein to grow larger, and eventually, becomes stronger and tougher. After it is healed, we were told and dialysis is needed, two needles are placed, one in the artery side, and one in the vein side of the fistula.

Plastic tubing attached to the needles connects one to the artificial kidney. With one needle placed to take the blood to the machine for cleansing, and the second needle to return the blood back to the body. The needles are left in until the treatment is finished, usually about three-four hours.

Doug went through the surgery well, but suffered a great amount of pain in his arm afterward. Now that the fistula was surgically placed, he would be playing a waiting game, worrying if the fistula would have time to heal before it was to be used.

Sooner Than Expected: On May 31, just six days after having his fistula surgery, I came home from shopping to find David and Doug sitting at the dining room table. Glancing at Doug, as I placed the grocery bag on the kitchen counter, I could sense that something was wrong.

"Are you all right Doug?" I asked, as he sat there resting his head in the palms of his hands.

"Not too good," he replied weakly.

"What's wrong?"

"I feel sick," he answered, in letting me know he had vomited a couple of times earlier.

"I almost vomited in the parking lot!" he exclaimed, when arriving at Dr. Baldinger's office that morning with David, whom had an eye appointment.

"I no sooner sat down in the waiting room," he continued, "that I had to get up and run straight to the bathroom to vomit. And I almost didn't make it there!" I could tell by the way he now looked, hollow-eyed with deep dark circles underneath, that he was much sicker than he thought.

"Did you call the doctor?"

"No!" he snapped. Of course not! I thought. He was to pick up his race car that afternoon.

Sick and needing dialysis sooner than expected, Doug was admitted to Potomac Hospital that day, making it his second admittance in six days time. Due to the fistula not healed, Dr. Bas had to perform surgery the next morning by making a temporary access for hemodialysis. In doing so, a Subclavian Vein Catheter would be surgically placed within Doug's upper chest area near his right shoulder. The thin catheter with two ports would be inserted into Doug's subclavian vein, where his entire blood supply would be shunted through this site to filter out impurities normally removed by the kidneys.

Muscular to begin with, Doug had developed his muscles even more so by all the heavy lifting required on his previous job. Which, during the time of the procedure, Dr. Bas had a difficult time trying to insert the catheter within Doug's shoulder muscle. Having a strong pain tolerance, Doug found this hard to bear by given just a local for pain.

As I sat there watching him, in pure agony, that morning as the doctor tried time after time to insert the catheter, I could tell it was all beginning to get the best of him. You could see it in his eyes. "I'm sorry Doug," the doctor said as he tugged forth, knowing the pain he was causing him. "Please bear with me."

After the procedure Dr. Bas explained to Doug, that the area he had to get to was not easy. "Making it hard," he said, "due to your large muscle size."

When and where does it all end? I thought, as the doctor departed.

How much more can Doug take?

How much more can I take? In having to watch him suffer so.

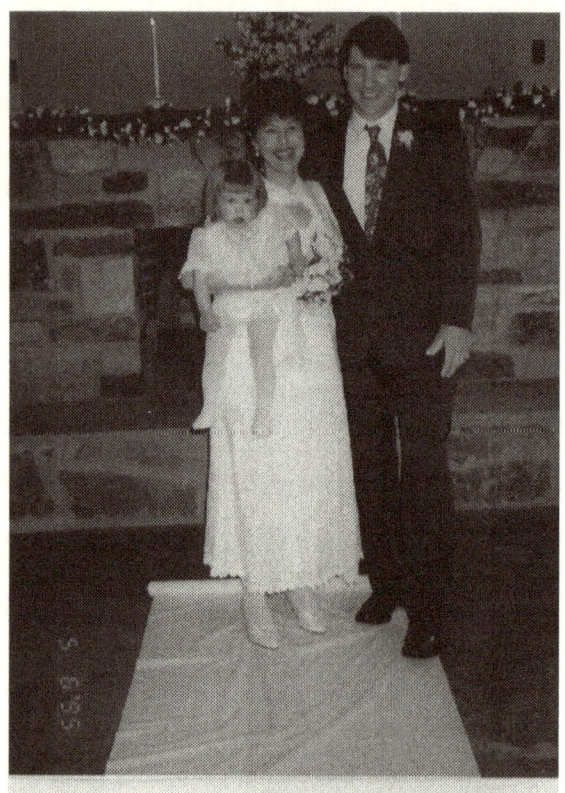

Doug and Sharon holding Melissa
age 21 months on their wedding
day, May 6, 1996.

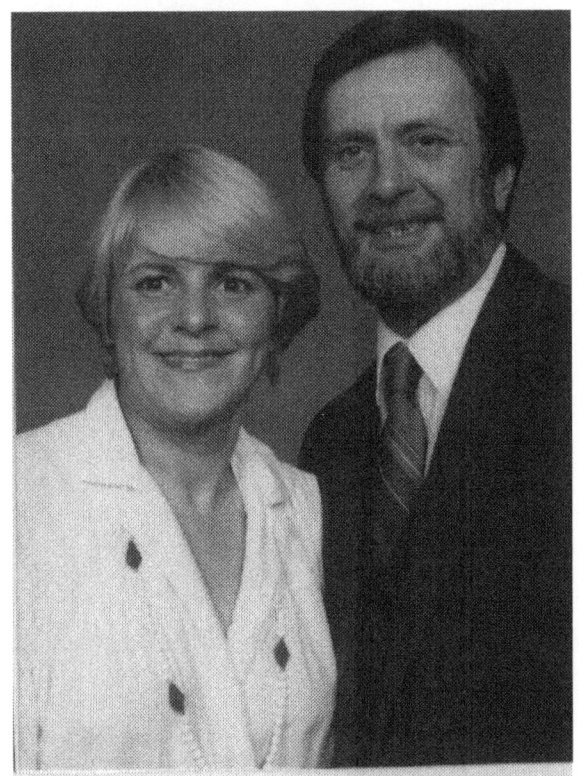

Uncle Alan and Aunt Carole, former
owners of Alan's Coffee Service

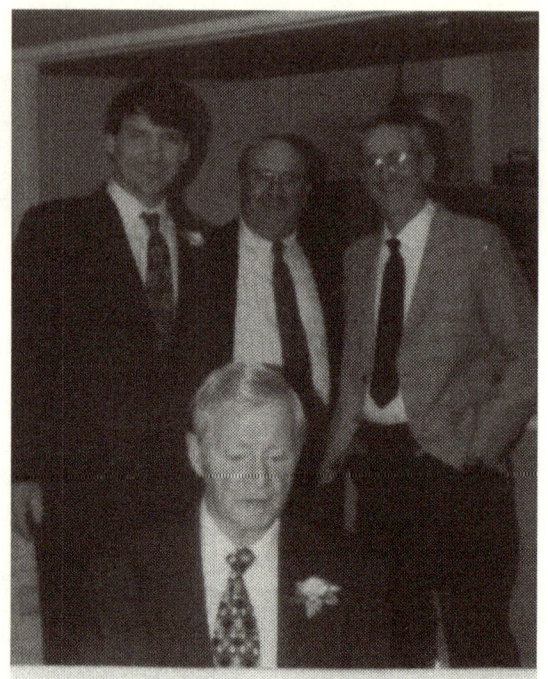

Doug with neighbor & racing
buddy, George Exline, Dad
(Vic) and Father-in-Law,
Don Burlew at Doug &
Sharon's Wedding,
May 6, 1995

CHAPTER 8

DIALYSIS TREATMENT * DIET

Late that same afternoon on June 1, 1995, Doug was given his first dialysis treatment at Potomac Hospital. The first two treatments were given on short intervals, with the second one given on the following day to which he was discharged afterward. Sent home with tape placed over the thin catheter tube that was left embedded, he was told to return three days later to the Continental Dialysis Center located less than five minutes from home.

It was there that he took his dialysis treatments three to three-and-a-half hours a day, three times a week. Waiting for the fistula to heal, he continued taking his treatments through the catheter in his upper chest for four weeks. The procedure was painless for him as it was connected directly to the in-placed catheter. However, the catheter was bothersome at times, by having to prevent it from getting wet when showering, as well as having to be extra careful not to disturb it during the day and while sleeping, for fear it would come out. Happy to be rid of the catheter within time, he was now overwhelmed by the size of the extra large dialysis needles that had to be placed into his fistula prior to treatment. Having to endure the painful connection, he dreaded further treatment.

Diet: Being on dialysis, Doug had to be on a special diet - an important part of treatment for Chronic Kidney disease. When the kidneys can no longer remove wastes and excess fluids from the body, fluids and certain foods have to be limited. This reduces the build-up of harmful poisons in the blood between treatments.

Doug accepted his limited diet, but was not all that happy about it. Giving up some of his favorite foods, such as: tomatoes, bananas, cantaloupe, potatoes, peanut butter, beans, and the amount of liquids he could have, upset him. The following topics are reasons why a 'special diet' is required due to kidney disease.

Protein: Your body needs protein for growth, building muscles, healing tissues, and for fighting infections and illness. When you have kidney disease, the amount of protein you eat must be controlled.

There are two types of protein to be aware of: "high quality" and "low quality." High quality proteins include meat, fish, chicken, turkey, dairy products and eggs. Low quality proteins are found in foods such as vegetables, bread, cereals and fruit.

When protein is digested and used by the body, it leaves behind a waste product called UREA. When the kidneys do not work properly, urea stays in the blood. This can cause nausea, vomiting, hiccups, and can make you feel weak and tired.

Dialysis and Diet help to alleviate these symptoms, because they both help to keep the level of urea down. However, as your body needs some protein to function, once you are on dialysis some protein intake is necessary.

Potassium: Potassium is a mineral found in all fresh fruits, vegetables, milk, chocolate and nuts. It is necessary for life because it is important to the health of all nerves and muscles, including the heart. However, too much or too little can be dangerous for the heart, as high levels of this mineral can even cause death.

There are usually no warning signs of high potassium levels, so therefore, if the potassium becomes too high, it can affect your heart by causing irregularities, and arrhythmias that could lead to heart failure. Doug, a hearty fruit and vegetable eater, was dishearten having to watch his potassium intake.

Sodium: The kidneys usually remove extra sodium. If your kidneys are not working normally, sodium will build up in the body. The body will hold fluids, causing weight gain and high blood pressure. Therefore, Doug had to watch his salt intake, primarily due to his already elevated blood pressure.

Fluids: Fluids are usually limited in a kidney patient's diet. An exception being made only if the patient has not started dialysis, whereas, Potassium and Fluids do not have to be watched very closely.

The kidneys use fluids, in the form of urine to get rid of waste products. If your kidneys are not working properly, the fluid stays in the body. Increased fluid in the body increases the risk of stroke and heart damage. Because of the increased risks, the amount of fluids you may have each day will be restricted.

Doug was informed that thirst was not a good way to decide on how much he wanted to drink, therefore, he was given an exact fluid allowance he could do so per day. Often thirsty, his drinking was one of the most difficult things he had to contend with. Being used to drinking as much as he wanted, he was now having to sip on limited amounts – never quite satisfying his thirst.

Phosphorous: Phosphorous is one of the building blocks of bone and is found in large amounts of dairy products, nuts, and dried beans and peas. When the kidneys are not able to remove excess phosphorus from the body, it builds up in the blood and tissues and can pull calcium from the bones. This will make bones weak and cause them to break easily. Due to Doug being on dialysis and a limited diet, he had to take several antacid/calcium supplement tablets per day to prevent bone loss.

CHAPTER 9

WHAT IS DIALYSIS?

Dialysis is a process, which uses either a machine or a special fluid installed into the peritoneal cavity, to help clean and filter the blood, just like a healthy kidney would. There are two types of dialysis: Hemodialysis and Peritoneal Dialysis. The following will give an insight on what options we had pertaining to treatment when Doug was first diagnosed with End Stage Renal Disease.

Hemodialysis: With hemodialysis, an artificial kidney (hemodialyzer) is used to cleanse the blood. During a hemodialysis treatment, the patient's blood is passed through tubing into a machine, which contains the artificial kidney. After wastes and extra fluids are taken out of the blood, the blood flows back through the tubing and into the body.

Inside the machine, there are two compartments. One compartment holds the patient's blood and the other holds a special cleaning fluid called Dialysate. A thin membrane made of cellophane, or a similar material, which has thousands of tiny holes, separates the two compartments. Blood cells and other important substances in the blood remain in one compartment because they are too large to pass through the holes in the cellophane membrane. However, the smaller waste products and excess water can pass through the membrane and are washed away by the dialysate.

For most people, hemodialysis treatments are needed three times a week. The procedure is done at an outpatient dialysis unit or home. Many units allow patients to arrange their treatment around their work, school or family schedules. If dialyzing at home, special training is needed for the patient and his/her treatment partner.

High-Flux Hemodialysis is a fairly new technique. It speeds up dialysis by the use of more permeable dialysis membranes and increases blood flow through the machine. In general, treatment time can be reduced with this new procedure. Not all patients are suited for this treatment, especially those with low blood pressure and those who cannot control their fluid intake.

Some side effects may occur from hemodialysis. This is usually caused by the rapid changes in the body's fluid and chemical balance during treatment. Two major side effects are muscle cramps (similar to a "charlie-horse") and hypotension (a sudden drop in blood pressure).

Symptoms of hypotension start with dizziness and may lead to an upset stomach and perhaps vomiting. Both muscle cramps and hypotension are more common when a patient first starts dialysis, of if he/she has not followed the proper diet between treatments. These side effects can often be treated quickly and easily with no complications.

Peritoneal Dialysis: In this type of dialysis, the cleaning process takes place inside the peritoneal cavity rather than passing through a machine.

Peritoneal dialysis gets its name from the Peritoneum. The peritoneum is a thin membrane that stretches around the internal organs in the body. During dialysis, the peritoneum does the same job that the membrane of the artificial kidney does during hemodialysis. That is, it acts as a filter that allows wastes to be removed by the blood.

To perform peritoneal dialysis, a small soft catheter is surgically placed into the abdomen. A special dialysis solution is passed through the catheter and into the abdominal cavity, which is the space next to the peritoneum. While this solution is in the abdominal cavity, it cleans the blood that passes through the peritoneum. The sugar in the solution acts like a magnet and draws water and wastes through the peritoneum and into the solution.

Just like the membrane in the kidney machine, the openings or pores in the peritoneum are so small that only the waste products can pass through; the blood continues to circulate throughout the body. After a certain period of time, the dialysis solution is drained from the abdomen, taking the wastes from the blood with it.

There are three different ways one can perform peritoneal dialysis: **Continuous Ambulatory Peritoneal Dialysis (CAPD)** is a self-care form of peritoneal dialysis, which is performed by the patient at home. CAPD allows the patient more freedom since no machine is needed to perform CAPD.

With CAPD, the dialysate solution is passed from a special plastic bag into the abdominal cavity. It stays there for four-six hours. The dialysate is then drained back into the bag and fresh solution is replaced in the abdomen. The entire process takes 30-40 minutes and most people change their solution four times a day. The solution can be changed in any clean, well-lit, private place.

Continuous Cycler Peritoneal Dialysis (CCPD) This type of dialysis is the same as **CAPD** except that: a) it is done with a machine and b) it is done during the night while the patient sleeps. In this method, a machine called a cycler is connected to the catheter, and it continuously fills and drains the dialysate from the abdominal cavity throughout the night.

Intermittent Peritoneal Dialysis: (IPD) This type of dialysis can be done at home or in the hospital. With IPD, treatments are several times a week, with a session lasting 10-12 hours. The same type of cycler used in CCPD is used to add and drain the dialysate.

Complications of Peritoneal Dialysis: A major problem that can occur with peritoneal dialysis is Peritonitis or infection of the peritoneum. This happens when the opening where the catheter enters the body becomes infected or when there is a problem in connecting or disconnecting the catheter from the bags. The chance of getting peritonitis can be reduced if the patient follows the procedure outlined by the physician or nurse.

Doug selected hemodialysis for his choice of dialysis treatment. It seemed more reasonable and less complicated to him. Having received treatments after a brief time, he began to go downhill some. Although he had more strength than most patients after treatment, his biggest downfall was feeling so tired. Something he was not quite used to.

Feeling Helpless: Doctor Greenspan informed Doug before going on dialysis, that he might be a candidate for a kidney transplant. I remember that day as if it were yesterday. On one of our visits to Dr. Greenspan, Doug asked the doctor what would happen if his creatinine kept going up. A terrible fear began to overtake me as the doctor discussed the probabilities of dialysis or transplantation. Glancing at Doug as the doctor spoke, I could see the color slowly drain from his face, in now knowing the full seriousness of his health.

Emotionally Overwhelmed: Like always, Dr. Greenspan's nurse, Delores, did Doug's blood work before leaving the office. While doing so, she would joke and tease with him, something they each did. He not only cut-up with Delores, but with all his nurses - making their day as well as his.

As they kidded back and forth, I noticed a wall shelf that contained pamphlets on kidneys and transplants. Getting permission, I took a couple on the way out. While leafing through them later that evening,

I became emotionally overwhelmed to what I had read. Tears filled my eyes, knowing, what was yet to be. Why Lord? Why? I thought, as I sat there numb with grief. What did Doug do to deserve all this? I wanted to hide the pamphlets, so he could not see them. I did not want him to know what all was involved. It was all so hard for me to grasp, I thought. How would it be for him?

Even though Doug was a grown man, being the youngest, he was the baby of the family. I worried about him – for him, as I did for all my grown kids. I wanted to protect them from all evil, and of all the unknown consequences thereof. Sad, and mad all at the same time, I felt so helpless to what I could do.

I have come to the understanding, though, that perhaps the most difficult task for any person with a serious illness is the collection of enough understandable information from which we have to make difficult choices. In the case of worsening kidney disease, I have found, with its continuous downhill course, as well as the need to prepare for, and adjust to renal failure in an uncertain future, bring fear and sometimes terror to the diabetic patient and his family.

CHAPTER 10

GETTING READY FOR TRANSPLANT

Laura's Gift: Doug's youngest sister, Laura, knew the heartbreak her brother was going through. Being the sensitive, sincere person that she is, "out of love", offered one of her kidneys to him. Although Sharon and I offered to do the same, he chose his sister. Just thirteen months apart, he and Laura were very close, and in ways were somewhat alike.

Laura was always the fit one in the family. Eating all the right foods, jogging, walking, and keeping her weight just right. Young and trim looking, at 5-foot 10 inches tall and weighing 138-lbs, one would have never known she was the mother of Michael, a teenage son then.

Transplant Team: With Doug on dialysis less than three weeks, I made an appointment to meet with the transplant team at Fairfax Hospital to see if he would be a candidate for a transplant. Doug, Sharon, and I were a bit anxious as the three of us arrived that Tuesday morning on June 20, 1995. We were put to ease when greeted by Mrs. Pat DiSanto, a friendly Kidney Transplant Coordinator. We were ushered to a conference room and when seated, she wanted to know Doug's age and how long he had been on dialysis? The age he had become diabetic? If he was working and did he have health insurance?

We were also introduced to the Social Worker. "Who will advise you," Mrs. DiSanto said, "about Medicare, Medicaid, and other insurance coverage. As well as helping with any psychosocial and family matters if you need it."

In addition, we were to meet the Transplant surgeon who would explain the evaluation process and answer any questions that we may have had. "Having an evaluation," Mrs. DiSanto said, "does not commit one to going ahead with the operation, but merely giving you more information about our treatment options." "Before recommending a transplant," she continued, "your physician will carefully review: your overall health; how well you follow directions and take your prescribed medications, and your insurance coverage."

Types Of Donor Transplants: We were told there are three types of donor kidney transplants: A kidney from an unrelated, deceased person; a ("cadaver" transplant), A kidney from a living relative, and a kidney from an unrelated living person.

"Occasionally," Mrs. DiSanto said, "A person will receive a kidney from a living, but unrelated, individual, such as a spouse, in-law, or very close friend." "However," she informed, "more than half of all kidney recipients receive an organ from a deceased (cadaveric) donor." Then telling us, due to a shortage in donor organs, the waiting period for a suitable cadaveric kidney could take up to two years.

We were also informed if you were a Type 1 Diabetic, as Doug was, he might be able to receive the Combined Kidney/Pancreas

Transplantation. Nearly one-third of patients who have renal failure have diabetes as the cause, whereupon, some of these individuals may benefit from receiving a new pancreas at the same time as the kidney. Stating that, both organs are taken from a deceased (cadaver) donor.

"The surgery," Mrs. DiSanto said, "takes about two to four hours longer than with the kidney alone." Saying, that the hospital stay may also be a bit longer receiving the dual transplant. The advantages are many, we learned, by having the dual transplant, but the biggest one is no further need for insulin shots, along with preventing the long-term problems associated with diabetes (such as vision impairment and amputation.) We were informed as well, that the same medications used to prevent rejection of a kidney transplant are also used for kidney/pancreas transplant.

We were well advised that transplantation is a treatment option only. It is not a cure for end-stage renal disease. The transplantation advantages over dialysis make it an attractive option for many patients such as: freedom from reliance on dialysis; fewer dietary and fluid restrictions; better rehabilitation; overall better health and energy level.

Upon all information given, Doug did not change his mind on which donor selection he had chosen. "My sister is giving me one of her kidneys," he voiced proudly, in letting Mrs. DiSanto know. "I'm glad," he said, knowing the success rate for a living donor is greater than a cadaver." "Not only that," he remarked. "Due to a shortage in donor organs, the waiting period may take up to two years! Maybe longer. I don't wanna wait that long!"

Doug was anxious to have the transplant. Overwhelmed by what all had happened to him in the past and present, he was looking forward to his "new lease on life." He just wanted to feel better.

Compatibility: Respecting his decision, Mrs. DiSanto went on to inform the pros and cons being a donor. "If Laura is found healthy," she said, "donating a kidney will be of no harm to her." Also letting us know that Laura's recovery would be more rapid than Doug's, and that her continuing life with one kidney would not affect her health in any way. For your new kidney to work properly," she told Doug, "you and your sister's kidney must be "compatible."

To establish as close a match as possible, the recipient and the donor organ are evaluated for characteristics that indicate compatibility. To determine compatibility, blood types are compared using the following parameters: ABO compatibility, Human leukocyte antigens (HLA) antigen matching, and Cross-match compatibility. Because these antigens play an essential role in the immune system, they are used to determine compatibility between kidney donor and recipient.

Cross-Match is the compatibility between recipient and donor. In general, the more closely the donor and recipient "match," the greater it is for a successful transplant. We were told that everyone has at least six important antigens. If the donor's six antigens match those of the recipient it would be considered a "perfect match." Mrs. DiSanto expressed that the ideal kidney donor is an identical twin.

We were also informed that siblings have a greater chance of being a perfect match because they have the same parents, as a parent automatically shares at least three antigens with a child. Living donors are usually from the immediate family, a mother, father, sister, brother, or son or a daughter whom is at least 18-years-old, or they may be cousins, aunts, or uncles.

We were then given the choice of what hospital we wanted the transplant to take place, along with their success rate. With Fairfax Hospital, serving the Northern Virginia area in transplant surgery, with an excellent success rate, and just being a half-hour away, we chose to have it there.

We did not get to see the transplant surgeon that day because he was in surgery, but were told we could see him when Doug came back for his pre-transplant testing. We were further informed that Laura would be put through a series of tests too. Not only to reveal compatibility, but also, to determine if she was healthy enough.

"The evaluation may reveal certain conditions that need to be corrected before transplant surgery," Mrs. DiSanto advised. "In rare instances, the work-up may disclose a problem that makes transplantation ill-advised, and if so, the physician would outline another plan." All these tests you will be taking," she continued, "are conducted because the transplant team wants to do everything in its power to help ensure you a successful transplant."

We also talked with the social worker that day, who offered to help Doug find a future job. We had discussed how long he had been out of work due to his eye condition, and now, that he was on dialysis. "I can no longer do what I was doing." Doug told her, "because of the heavy lifting that's required." "Find what trade you want to get into," she answered, "and when you're able to work again, I'll try to help you find something."

Handling Major Costs: We also discussed health insurance. Doug informed her that he was on Sharon's work policy now that they were married. We were told different insurance policies cover all, part or none of the transplant surgery, including the three months of follow-up treatment. "It is also covered by Medicare, as is dialysis," the social worker informed us. Telling us that the two main ways to pay for these expenses are through private insurance and government programs such as (Medicare, Medicaid, and VA benefits).

We were told kidney failure is different from other major illnesses, and that patients with permanent kidney failure are eligible for Medicare benefits regardless of age, if they meet other eligibility requirements. Informing because of the high cost of treatment, Doug would be expected to sign up for Medicare even though he had private insurance.

"No single plan will be likely to meet your needs," she continued. "You will probably have to use some combination of two or three of them." Laura did not need insurance we were told, as all living donor's hospitalization is covered by the recipient's insurance.

Our social worker then touched on our personal feelings. "It's natural to be concerned," she said. "If you feel depressed or uneasy, talk it out! I'm here to answer any questions. To ease your fears and to help you cope." As Doug sat there with head hung, one could see that he was very tired and weary. After all, he had been struggling with mixed emotions for sometime. But as for help, he did not feel he needed any. Saying, "I have my family. They are there for me!"

As for Sharon, she had mixed feelings. Although she was a cheerful, lively person, she had a hard time dealing with stressful situations. With all Doug's problems, her life crumbled right along with his. I'll never forget just week's prior, when she first found out that Doug would be going on dialysis. I was preparing dinner that evening when she came by from work. As soon as she entered the kitchen I could tell she had been crying.

"I had no idea Doug's condition was that bad!" she told me, being confused and upset over the unexpected suddenness of his diagnosis.

"Having to work, I didn't get to go with him when he had his appointments, so I never knew what was being said."

"Although I would hear ya' all discussing about it," she said sadly, "I just didn't think it was that serious!

"We've only been married three weeks," she said, with tear filled eyes. Sharon was totally disheartened, and in a somewhat state-of-shock to it all. She could deal with Doug's diabetes, but had a difficult time adjusting to his kidney problem. Although there was a lot of strain and pressure put on her, through it all, she stuck by her man. She strived hard to make matters better for him.

We had no idea that Sharon was not aware of how bad Doug's kidneys were. Even though we knew, it was still a shock to us as well. I knew the heartache she was going through, as it was for us too.

With a heavy heart, and tear-stung eyes when the social worker asked my feelings that afternoon, my only reply was, "I wish his pain was my pain. I wish it were me." Having discussed all issues and upon leaving, we were told the appointments would be set up right away for Doug and Laura to be evaluated, with Doug being sent to the lab that very day for blood work.

Pre-Transplant Testing: To determine Doug's compatibility, eighteen tubes of blood were taken to test his blood count, blood and tissue type, blood chemistries, and immune system function. At such a time, he was told, contacting hepatitis could be serious in kidney transplant patients and to protect those who have not been exposed, he was given his first hepatitis C injection out of three.

Within a week, Laura went through the same ordeal as Doug - eighteen tubes of blood taken to determine her donor compatibility. Over a two-week period they each had chest x-rays, electrocardiogram (EKG), as well as an echocardiogram with ultrahigh frequency sound waves used to look at the heart. This was all followed by a sonogram, which creates a picture of your kidneys and surrounding structures.

They each had to do a 48-hour urinalysis, where they collected their urine in a plastic jug container, and took it everywhere they went during that time. In addition, they each were given physiological testing - the study of the function of tissues and organs.

Doug was given a stress test, an exercise session to measure the strength of his heart. He also had a heart arteriogram, an x-ray of the arteries taken by dye through the arm. Laura was given a kidney arteriogram, whereupon, the dye was injected into the top inner-side of her thigh. The process, having this done, was somewhat more difficult than Doug's, by having to inject a sizeable needle into a jugular vain. After the procedure, she had to remain flat on her back for four hours - a precaution to prevent further bleeding.

Using the restroom when her time was up, she discovered that she was still bleeding. Therefore, she had to endure another four hours on her back before leaving. At which time, she was told to continue the duration for the next 24 hours at home. Doug had taken Laura to the hospital that morning, staying by her side throughout the day. More impatient than Laura after their ten-hour ordeal, he said, "It's the least I can do for all she's doing for me!"

A Match: Within a week, all test results came back. Giving them a good overall health report, along with the good news that Laura had three antigens that matched those of Doug's. We were ecstatic! Our next step would be setting up an appointment for the transplant.

In mid-July, Mrs. DiSanto introduced Doug, Laura and I to Dr. Johann Jonsson, the transplant doctor, whom was the Director of the Kidney/Pancreas Transplant Services. Dr. Jonsson, a gentle, soft-spoken, middle-aged man, greeted us with a warm smile. Once we were in his office, he began right away with all the pros and cons we should know about the upcoming transplant.

First, and above all, Dr. Jonsson wanted Doug to realize the seriousness and the importance of taking transplant medication. Explaining to him that in addition to medications he would ordinarily need, he would also be given potent immunosuppressive drugs to treat transplant rejection. "These anti-rejection drugs," he stressed, "helps to keep your immune system from rejecting your new kidney."

He also informed us that the medications could cause side effects, which tend to diminish as the doses are decreased. "In time they do," he said. "In fact, so much so that you may feel you no longer need them." Again, he expressed the importance of the anti-rejection medication, by saying, "For each day you would miss taking your medication, you would be losing valuable life span to your new kidney." At which time Doug assured Dr. Jonsson, he would have no problem taking his medications. He said that the kidney his sister was giving him was a special gift, and he was going to take good care of it.

Transplant Procedure: Having no misunderstandings about the importance of transplant medications, Dr. Jonsson continued by giving him details of the transplant procedure. Telling Doug, that he would be making an incision 8 to 10 inches long above the groin. "We (the surgical team) will attach the artery and vein of your new kidney," he said, "to one of your arteries and veins." He also informed him that they would attach the new kidney's ureter (tube that carries urine to the bladder) to his bladder.

We were also told that Doug's own kidneys would not be removed. Saying the new kidney would be implanted in front of his abdomen with it being easier to connect to the bladder. "Sometimes the new kidney begins making urine during the operation," Dr. Jonsson said. "Whereas at times, it takes up to two or three weeks to do so. We've seen this happen both ways several times. In case of it not working," he said, "one has to go on dialysis until kidney function takes place."

Concluding with Doug, Dr. Jonsson informed us that the surgery would take approximately four to six hours. Saying that the length of his hospital stay would depend on his progress after surgery, with the average seven to ten days. Focusing on Laura, the doctor asked if she had any questions or anything she wanted to know before surgery took place.

Laura's Concern: There was one issue that worried Laura, which was not discussed and that was Doug's racing. If he continued to race, she thought, what chance would there be in him injuring his new kidney? Laura had previously discussed this issue with Mrs. DiSanto, and it was she, that now reminded her of it. Laura was giving up one of her kidneys; therefore, she had plenty of reason to worry for not wanting Doug to take risk. For fear, he would lose his kidney and have to go through it all again.

"I see no reason why he couldn't continue racing," the doctor said smiling. He dampened the situation when he went on to say, "If you can race without having any accidents, I see no problem." Informing him that the new kidney would be placed in front of the abdomen where it's not quite as protected, as it would be in the back. Reminding him then of what Doug said prior, "The kidney your sister is giving you is a very valued gift."

When racing one has no guarantee of never having accidents. Wrecks are just a part of it. And Lord knows, Doug had had his share. Racing was a hobby that he loved and was very good at, but now, it did not seem quite as important to him. Respecting Laura's concern, he agreed to give it up. He knew the kidney she was about to give him, was, and would be, a valued gift – the gift of life. A gift that would free him from dialysis - giving him a new "lease on life."

With all tests and discussions resolved, Doug and Laura planned their transplant for October, three months away. They were told to call the transplant center six weeks prior, so they could schedule the date.

New Home: Shortly after the final plans were made for the transplant, Doug, Sharon, and Melissa moved into their new home. In the same neighborhood they'd rented, and within a short walking distance from where Doug grew up. The home they had bought was restored as a new one; in having had fire damages a couple of year's prior. A beautiful home, that sat on a grassy knob, overlooking thirty-two-year old homes in the neighborhood. The houses being the same age as Doug then!

Doug and Sharon seemed much happier now that things were looking up for them, everything was a lot less complicated than it had been. They were finally settled in their beautiful home, and were looking forward to brighter days.

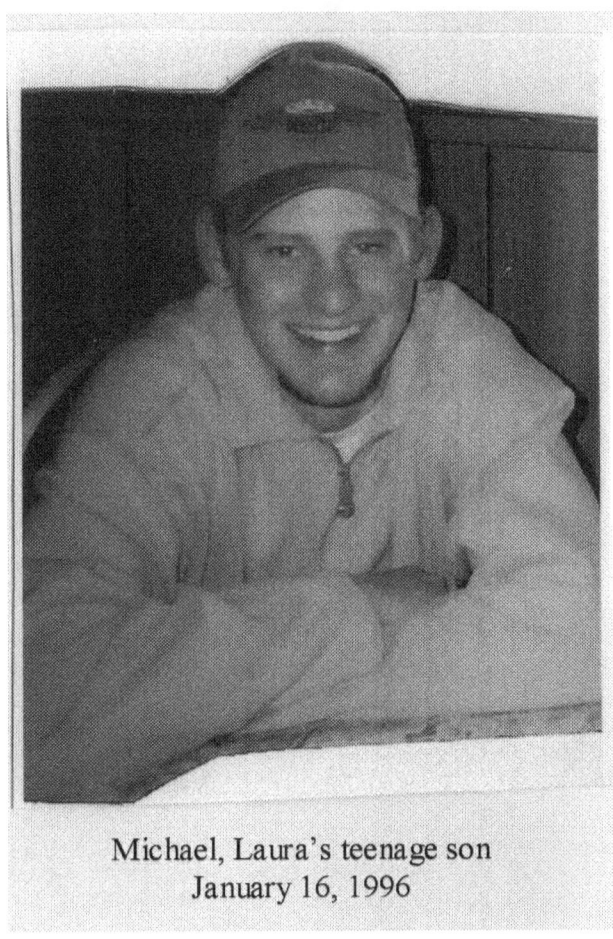

Michael, Laura's teenage son
January 16, 1996

CHAPTER 11

DISAPPOINTING NEWS

Postponed: In late August, just weeks shy from setting their transplant date, Doug received disappointing news from Laura. "We can't have the transplant as planned," she told him. She had to go through training on conversion software due to a changeover at work, for then, Virginia First Mortgage, and there was no way she could take six weeks off as the doctor stated. Then explained that being divorced, single, and having just received a new job promotion, she could not afford to sacrifice her employment during that time. "We'll have to postpone!" she told Doug. "Until the end of December, or maybe, until the first of the year." The news of the postponement was devastating to him.

The Waiting: Never having problems with needles in the past, Doug was now finding it quite difficult to cope with the extremely large dialysis needles that had to be inserted into his forearm three times a week. He was disappointed that he would have to continue this regiment, as well as not able to drink what he wanted, nor eat the foods he loved.

Knowing the disappointments and difficulties Doug was now going through, to help pass time, the family made every effort possible to go by the dialysis center to visit him during treatment time. Having a dislike for needles anyway, David found his one and only trip very upsetting. Watching the dialysis procedure overwhelmed David, whereas, one of the nurses seeing him pale looking, asked Doug if his brother was all right.

"I wasn't feeling all that well when I went there," David later recalled. Saying, watching the dialysis procedure didn't help him any. "Poor Doug," he'd said, "I don't know how he stands it!"

Turned Down: That particular occasion made me remember the time he and Margie wanted to take out a life insurance policy. Doing so, a Health Representative came by their house one evening to do blood work on David. After the procedure, he became very weak and dizzy. Feeling like he might faint, he placed his head on the dining room table. He was so upset with himself, saying later, "I shouldn't have watched. I could feel myself getting weaker and weaker."

David tried so hard to keep his blood sugar controlled at work, knowing, he would be having the blood test that evening. Thinking that he had done a good job, he still revealed a mild elevated sugar reading at the time the test was taken. Denied by the insurance company because of this, David felt hurt and rejected in being deprived of something he thought was uncalled for. "I could see being denied if my sugar was extremely high," he had told us afterward. "It just isn't fair," he said, thinking he was denied because he was a diabetic.

David was beside himself, since he knew his blood sugar was normal when they came for the test. Voicing his opinion over the matter, he was informed they would take him, but only on a smoker's rate. Having never smoked, he rejected the policy, as he was not about to pay an extra high rate for something he had never done.

International Speedway: Being on dialysis had not stopped Doug's love for racing. Knowing he could no longer do this after his transplant gave him that much more incentive to do so. He would cherish the next few races with his now owned modified race car.

Doug would be given the opportunity to drive his modified two weekends at Richmond International Speedway. He was anxious to return, as he had been there once before when the Doyles had owned the race car. This was a special event for him, to be able to race on an International Speedway to whom the 'Big Boys', NASCAR drivers were only allowed. It was a big attraction each year in October for the State Fair, whose fairgrounds are located adjacent to the racetrack.

The first weekend Doug qualified eighteenth and finished ninth – thrilled that he had finished in the top-10. Having made some changes to his car the second weekend, he was not as lucky, by not qualifying well enough to make the field. Not racing and knowing it would have been his last race ever, left him highly agitated and downhearted for a long time.

Having To Wait: Adding to Doug's misery, the following month in late November, Laura called to say they would have to reschedule their plans for the transplant again. "With the change over involving a work load on me," she announced, "we'll have to do it in April, instead as planned in late December or first of January." "You're kiddin!" Doug replied, surprised. Which, he did not take lightly.

During this time Doug was not feeling well, with his health deteriorating little by little each day. He and Sharon discussed the situation, which led them to believe that Laura was having second thoughts. As in the past, Sharon was willing to donate one of her kidneys. And with neither wanting to prolong the transplant any longer, she called the transplant center to see if she could be tested. Knowing about the delay and with Laura still planning to donate her kidney, the Coordinator told her it would be an expense for unnecessary tests done. Words cannot express how Doug felt when hearing this. He just knew he would never get a kidney!

When Laura called her transplant coordinator about the delay, she was told that Doug's condition was not life threatening and that the transplant could wait. With Doug double-checking Laura, she promised him she was not backing out.

"I'm going to do it!" she said.

"But you'll have to wait until I have the time.

"I can't jeopardize my job," she told him.

"I need to get things up and running!" Although Doug was scared, he knew he would have to wait – having to rely on his sister's faith.

Blizzard: With Christmas coming on, Doug was kept busy — which helped to occupy his time and mind. Not doing well as time went on, he kept reminding us how many more days it would be until the transplant. By the time Christmas arrived, one could tell dialysis was getting the best of him. Deprived of strength and energy, he had become weak and thin, with dark rings circling his sunken eyes.

The following month on January 6, 1996, Virginia had a severe snowstorm that nearly paralyzed the whole East Coast. It came in with a bang, dropping 18 inches of snow. The immediate concern during this time in the Washington Metropolitan area was getting all personnel and Dialysis patient's to their treatment center. Stating, it was a matter of life and death if patients went three or four days without treatment. To help get staff worker's and patients to their treatment center, the newscasters were asking for volunteers with 4-wheel-drives.

Having a four-wheel-drive and living less than five minutes from the Dialysis Center, Doug's only concern about getting to the treatment center was the personnel that worked there. He dreaded the thought of the Dialysis Center not opening. With his last treatment on Friday of that week, and with the storm coming over the weekend, it seemed almost impossible that he'd be able to make his regular scheduled treatment for Monday, the next day. With ankles already swollen, he worried if he did not have treatment on time, he could develop poison toxins in his bloodstream.

Luckily, with the aid of volunteers, the Dialysis Center opened Monday, in late afternoon. With it such an enormous storm, the following days were just as hectic. Owning a four-wheel-drive and knowing the seriousness of Dialysis treatment and further need for transportation, Doug helped by taking patients to and from the Dialysis Center even though he was not feeling well himself.

CHAPTER 12

PREPARING FOR TRANSPLANT

Laura's Surprise: In the latter part of January, I decided to re-wallpaper our living room. This job being way overdo, I felt, would keep me busy in not thinking about the upcoming transplant. It was hard enough accepting one child's surgery, let alone two.

The job I undertook was a big one, because I had to strip the old wallpaper, prepare the wall, and put up new wallpaper. While preparing a wall one afternoon, Laura came rushing through the front door.

"Have you talked to Doug?" she asked, with a big smile on her face.

"No! What's up?"

"Doug didn't call?"

"No!" I answered. "What's wrong?"

"We can have the transplant now!" she exclaimed, all excited.

"You can what?" I answered, totally surprised by the suddenness of it all.

"My boss came in my office this morning and told me to go on with the transplant now. They hired temporary help to handle my work load until I can go back," she announced cheerfully.

I had mixed emotions when hearing the news. I was excited for them, but to put it bluntly, I was not ready for all this now! The entire time she was informing me I was looking at my walls. Only half of my wallpaper was down. What a mess I had!

"Aren't you excited for us?" she asked, sadly.

"Of course I am!" I replied.

"But look at my walls. They're only half done!"

"We have to set the date yet," she remarked, laughing.

"Maybe you'll have it finished by then. If not, just hire someone!" Doug called soon after and words cannot express the excitement in his voice.

"I would've called before this," he announced, "but I called the hospital right after Laura called."

"Mom," he said, being surprised, "I couldn't believe it!"

"I even asked her, "Are you sure about this Laura?" He had been excited twice before, only to be let down by having to postpone. Now knowing for sure they would be going through with it, he was ecstatic!

When he called the transplant center that afternoon, they told him it was his lucky day. Having had a cancellation, they set the date for February 8, just two weeks away! Hearing this, we immediately went into action. While Doug was counting how many more days he had on dialysis, and making appointments for he and Laura to have additional blood work done to make sure they were still compatible, I was getting an estimate on having my wallpapering done.

Laura's Birthday Party: On February 5, 1996, just three days prior to their scheduled transplant, the family celebrated Laura's 34th birthday. I prepared her favorite dinner, chicken and dumplings, along with her favorite cake – white with white frosting. It was an "extra" special occasion for us. With our main topic of conversation on the upcoming transplant – our spirits soared high!

Although we did not have their latest test back for the go-ahead yet, we still could not help but be excited. However, with it being seven months since they had the first one, the thought of their recent blood work not showing compatibility laid heavy on our minds. Things could change! Being notified of the results the day after Laura's birthday took a load off us, knowing their blood work stayed the same and the transplant would be as scheduled.

On the eve of their transplant, the entire family gathered to discuss the following morning's plans. Excited and anxious all at the same time, we laughed, joked, and had a good ol' time. Overly excited and wound-up, none of us got much rest that night. It seemed we had no sooner went to bed that it was time to get up.

Morning of Transplant: The following morning on the 8th was a nasty one. It was rainy, cold and damp. We certainly didn't complain - just thankful it wasn't snow. With it such a miserable morning, the traffic moved with ease getting us there much earlier than expected. On arriving, Doug and Laura signed in. While waiting to be called, after all paperwork was completed, Doug and Laura laughed and talked. It was hard to tell which one was the most excited.

Around 6:30 that morning, Doug and Laura's coordinators, Mrs. DiSanto and Mrs. Robinson greeted us with a big smile. They were our advisors, as they were the ones that coordinated all of the events, and to whom would keep us up to date throughout the day on the progress of their transplant.

They informed us that Doug and Laura would be taken to the pre-op room where they would be prepared for surgery. Once they were settled, we were told that Sharon, Laura's son, Michael, Vic and I could come in to see them before they were taken to surgery. Before leaving the waiting room, the entire family showered them with hugs and kisses and wished them the best of luck. They were whisked away then, to begin what we thought, and should have been, an uncomplicated ordeal. Unfortunately, it would turn out to be one of Doug's greatest nightmares. He says to this very day, "It's one I'd never want to go through again!"

Entering the pre-op room, we found Doug and Laura lying side by side on separate gurneys. At which time both were in the process of getting their IV's. With Doug's surgery more extensive and more complicated than Laura's, he had a more difficult time getting his IV than her by having to painfully undergo a greater needle preparation. Doug who had recently had a big smile, and whom was once cheerful, was now grim and solemn as the medical staff tried time after time to insert large sizable needles into his upper forearm. With blood soaked sheets and his wrenching face, one could tell the pain he was going through.

After an endless time they finally succeeded, saying, the difficult time they had was due to the veins moving. "Are you all right?" I asked, knowing what he had just went through. "Yeah," he muttered disgustedly, through clenched teeth with eyes closed. This isn't a good start! I thought. His once happy mood had now turned bleak.

"I Love Ya' Man": With Laura's surgery first, a nurse arrived from O.R. at 7:45 that morning to take her. Through tear-filled eyes as we knelt to kiss her and wish her luck, we were overwhelmed with love and pride, knowing she would be giving her brother a "New Lease on Life." Grinning ear to ear as they wheeled her out, she turned to Doug and said, "I love ya' man."

The attending nurse finding this quite funny and amusing, said, laughing, "I love ya' man – just don't take my Bud! Huh?" We all laughed with her quoting from the 'then' popular Budweiser commercial. It made our day by lifting tension and giving us something to talk about. As for the nurse, we are sure she still remembers the incident.

Around 8:00 A.M., their scheduled transplant time, they came from O.R. to get Doug. As we embraced him and wished him luck, he was not as good-humored as Laura when she went. With eyes closed, he didn't have much to say. The preparation for Doug's transplant had got the best of him, before his surgery ever began.

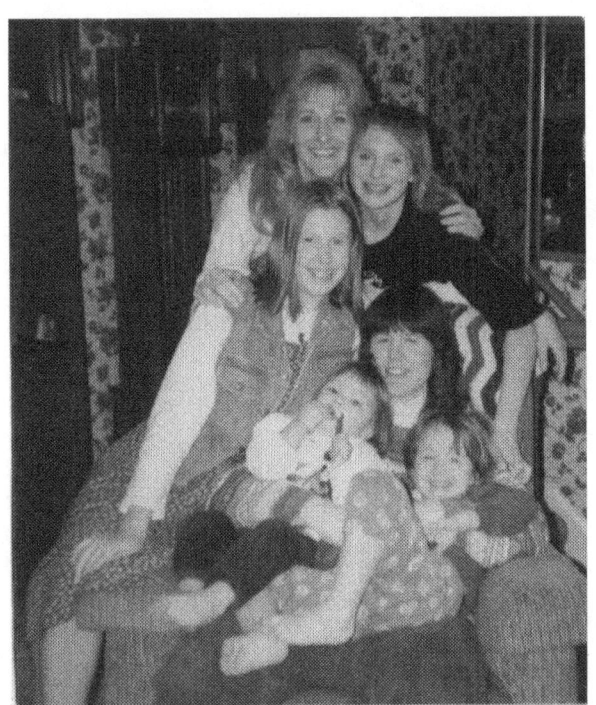

Laura on her 34th birthday (3 days prior to transplant) with neices, Jenny, Jessie, Melissa, sister Vicky and her daughter, Cari (other daughter Leah not pictured), February 5, 1996

CHAPTER 13

TRANSPLANT

Anxiously Waiting: With both, Laura and Doug gone, we were told to have breakfast if we had not had any. They told us to wait afterward in the main lobby, whereupon, we would be kept informed. After having had breakfast which Bobbi Stackhouse, a close friend, had treated us to, we went straight to the hospital chapel. Accompanied by a chapel priest there, a prayer was said in Doug and Laura's behalf that gave us inner-peace. Afterward, we went to the hospital lounge where we eagerly waited for an update on their progress. The transplant coordinators kept us informed throughout the morning, which helped to keep our anxieties at bay.

Approximately 1:30 that afternoon, we received word that Laura's surgery was over, and that she had been taken to the recovery room. "She's doing great!" they announced. What a relief it was to know it was all over and she was doing well. We could hardly wait to see her! We were still concerned, though. We had one more to go - anxiously waiting word about Doug.

Being restless, I went outside to get some fresh air. Not gone for long, I returned to find the family visibly upset. Asking if they had heard anything as yet, Vic answered, "Yes," but seemed hesitant in telling me anything. Looking at the family, I could tell by their expressions that something bad had gone wrong. Whereupon, I felt a sudden sickness come over me.

"They came down and told us the kidney wasn't working," Vic finally said, with his eyes glued to the floor.

"I thought they said that would be normal!" I exclaimed, with that possible.

"Mrs. DiSanto informed us," he said, "that normally the new kidney starts working right away!"

"She told us it wasn't uncommon for it not to work, but most cases it does."

"She referred to Doug's," he said, "as being a bit lazy."

"She'll keep us updated on his condition," he further informed. I was concerned hearing this, but relieved too. By the way everyone was acting at first, the thought had occurred to me that Doug took a turn for the worse. It was a blessing to know that all we had to deal with was just a lazy kidney. Thankful for his well-being, we each silently said a prayer and continued waiting for better news.

Laura's Surgery: Having surgery such as Laura's, a rib is removed to retrieve the donor's kidney. Laura's Urologist, Dr. Michael Hardy found that her kidney lay beneath the rib, so we were given the good news this was not done.

Although her surgery went well, Dr. Hardy encountered an unexpected situation that took surgery a little longer than expected. Due to her anatomy makeup in taking the left kidney, the smaller of the two, the doctor discovered additional blood vessels than normal. This made it more difficult and time consuming for him by having to connect and disconnect. Also, by not removing the rib, which is quite unusual with this type of surgery, it took a lot of time on his part to retrieve the full length of the main artery leading from the kidney. A procedure if not done properly, could cause problems for the transplant team reconnecting it to Doug.

Arriving to her room around 3:00 that afternoon, we did not know what to expect when first seeing Laura. Although we had been informed she did fine, we still felt anxious. Peering into her room, we were amazed to see her sitting up, wide awake and smiling. We could not get over how good she looked. One would never guess by looking at her that she had just been through major surgery.

Having been kept well medicated, she did not suffer much pain. However, due to what little pain she did have and the medication she was on, she was not allowed anything to eat nor drink, including ice chips for four long days for fear of her getting sick. With her saying, "That was the hardest thing I went through!" To help keep her lips moist, she did have the pleasure of using swab-sticks. After a couple of days, with a steady regimen doing this, and being so hungry with nothing to eat, laughing, she commented, "They're starting to taste real good!"

During her hospital stay, Laura was quite popular. Gaining attention from family, friends and coworkers. She was everyone's hero! She received cards, flowers, balloons, and a beautiful bracelet from Doug's in-laws, Don and Nancy Burlew, which she treasures to this day.

Sentimental and somewhat shy, Laura felt embarrassed by all the attention. She said, "I'm just doing something that I'd want someone do for me if needed." Staying in the hospital just four days, she was released before Doug, as was expected.

Doug's Surgery: It was late afternoon around 4:00 p.m. when Doug's coordinator came and told us that his new kidney was functioning all right. "Slowly," she said, "but working," "It'll be awhile before you can see him, though," she informed. Saying with him under anesthesia longer than expected, due to Laura's surgery taking longer, and the delay of his kidney working, he would be in recovery for some time.

Shortly thereafter, Doctors, Jonsson and Shaver met us in the lounge to inform us of Doug's progress. They said that he and the new kidney were doing fine in spite of the setbacks. However, they did inform us they had a difficult time placing the new kidney. Telling us that since Doug was slim through the abdomen area, it caused less space to work with. Having inquired about the delay of the kidney working, both doctors did not seem all that concerned, other than saying sometimes it happens. Telling us that the delay did not mean the kidney was not a good one.

Although the doctors had a difficult time placing Doug's new kidney in the lower abdomen, it has been proven more beneficial. Placing the kidney in the pelvic region makes it easier to attach the blood vessels of the kidney to the iliac vessels in the pelvis. As well as the ureter in this position would be much shorter in length, thus enabling it to function more satisfactorily and less likely to deteriorate. All in all, making it the choice for a greater chance of the transplant functioning satisfactorily.

Another helpful benefit by placing the kidney in the lower abdomen is it is least invasive and makes the kidney more accessible for biopsy and treatment. This will become very beneficial to Doug in time, as he will have had more than his share of biopsy and treatment.

Doug's Recovery: Around 8:00 p.m. that night, we were told we could go see Doug. He was in a private intensive care room, due to needing special care for a day or so. It had been twelve hours since we last saw him, so we were just as anxious to see him, as we were with Laura. Sharon, Vic and I went first, as the hospital did not allow more than two or three in the room at any given time. As we gazed into his dimly-lit room, we saw the complete opposite of what we had seen with his sister.

Entering, we observed a large white, sterile looking room, somewhat cheerful for its purpose. With Doug's bed placed by a large window overlooking the brightly lit street that lay below. The room was very quiet other than sounds from pulsating machines that surrounded him, and the scurrying of busy nurses watching over him. Still under the effects of anesthesia, he was resting easy.

Tiptoeing slowly as we neared his bed, we could not believe all the tubes we were seeing. They were in both arms, neck, nose, and bladder. As well as a clear plastic mask placed over his mouth with a breathing tube attached down his throat. Everywhere you looked there seemed to be some kind of tube or machine connected to him. It was sad to see him so lifeless; yet happy too, knowing the surgery had been a success.

Although highly sedated, he did respond to us some. In letting him know that George was there to see him, he seemed to tense up. George Exline, whom is a long time friend, and our next-door neighbor for 33 years then, had watched Doug grow up right along with his kids. Their ties became even closer as Doug got older and became involved in racing. Being on Doug's pit crew for a year or so, George, in his early fifties, decided to race as well. They had even raced in the same class against each other!

"I don't want George to see me like this...just the family," Doug moaned, through closed eyes. He knew George was concerned and meant well, but he didn't want him to see him the way he was. Saying with him very groggy and not able to communicate well, he did not feel at ease with anyone other than the immediate family.

George was disappointed by Doug's request when we told him. "I'll just go in for a quick minute," he remarked, wanting Doug to know he had been there for him. It did not matter, though, who went in to see Doug that night. We later learned, he didn't remember much about any of us being there.

Late afternoon the next day, Doug was moved from the intensive care unit to a room next to Laura's, which made it convenient for us during visiting hours. Although they wanted the same room together, it was not allowed because they were the opposite sex.

Doug was not pleased he was placed in a semi-private room with his bed opposite to the window, as he enjoyed looking out. "It's so boring in here," he commented dishearteningly one day, with time passing slowly for him. "All I have to look at is that bare wall and clock!" he said.

Wanting to cheer his Mom up, Michael bought her a "big" smiley-face balloon. With Doug commenting, "At least she has something to look at!" With most items forbidden in his room due to being a transplant patient, I was told he could have a balloon. "It's nice to look up and see something other than that bare wall and clock!" he said, cheerfully, pleased that I had bought him one and placed it on the wall next to the clock. Not having much to smile about, it helped to brighten his day. I was pleased myself that it helped.

Doug did not smile nor talk much for the first couple of days after his surgery. In fact, he wasn't able to do much of anything. Connected to an IV, and the large, balky, neck catheter, that was left to keep an eye on his body fluid levels, he found it hard to move, as well trying to sleep. One of the many reasons he wasn't smiling was due to the urethral catheter, which he despised. This was very uncomfortable for him, but was needed, so they could keep a close watch on his urine output.

During this time, he had discovered his penis had swollen about four times its normal size. Freaking him out, he immediately called for a nurse. While waiting, a transplant nurse that needed information from him, walked into the room, to whom Doug thought was the nurse he had called for. Whereupon, an un-shy Doug threw his blanket back, and yelled, "What's wrong with this?"

"Oh.... wait! Haw.... haw.... I'll get your floor nurse for you!" she said totally astonished, as she turned and hurried out the door. Within minutes, the floor nurse appeared. "What's the problem?" she asked. When Doug threw the blanket back this time, the nurse casually informed, "It's nothing to be alarmed about," she said, making light of it. "The swelling is due to irritation caused by the prolonged use of the urethral catheter. It'll go down once the catheter is out," she told him smiling.

Medications: Beginning his medications through the IV the day of his surgery, he was now taking fifty-two pills a day. Ranging from the potent immunosuppressive drugs to prevent rejection to several other types of drugs. Such as: medication for blood pressure, fluid, blood clotting, stomach, thrust, constipation, and a multiple vitamin. In addition, he was also given antibiotics to prevent pneumonia and other infections. All these taken in a variety of size and color, to which he was told he had to learn each of them by sight and what they were used for.

He was also given medication to prevent cytomegalovirus CMV, a member of the herpes group of viruses. It commonly occurs in man and normally produces symptoms milder than the common cold. However, in individuals whose immune systems are lowered it can cause more severe effects.

"Don't get used to your wife giving you your medications," a transplant nurse later warned, "because she may not be around at all times when your medicine is due." "You need to know them," she stressed. Then, she told him of an incident about a man who had relied on his wife for his medication. "And when she died unexpectedly," she said, "he had no idea which ones to take, nor the time to take them." "I'm not saying that this might happen to your wife," she added, "but you should know what you're taking!" Doug was listening, but his mind at that time was elsewhere. Everything seemed so confusing to him then, but vowed he would later learn.

OCD: Although not medically diagnosed with OCD, (obsessive compulsive disorder) Doug does have this disorder. When things are not done right, or on time, he literally goes to pieces. Even as a kid, his brother, David, always shook his head when he compared his dresser drawers to Doug's. Clothes folded and neatly stacked, one would find it hard to believe how such a young person could keep things so orderly. Because of this disorder, it made things more difficult for Doug to cope with.

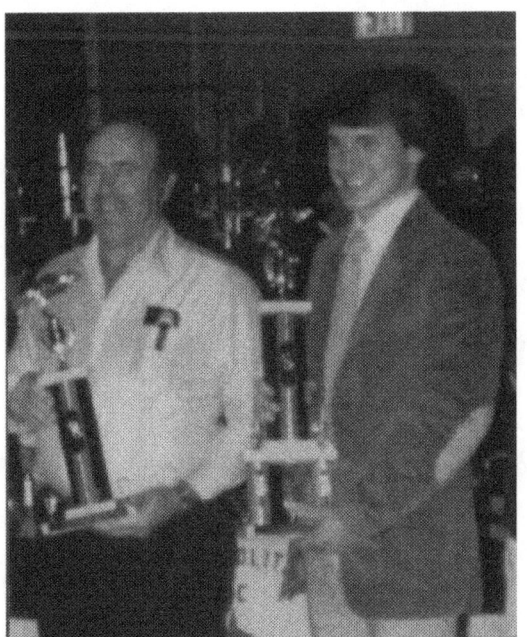

Doug with neighbor and
racing buddy, George Exline
with their trophies they
received in the Hobby class
at the MARF Banquet
(Metropolitan Auto Racing
Fans Club), November 1987.

CHAPTER 14

ADJUSTING * HUMAN-INTEREST STORY

High Blood Sugar: While in the hospital, Doug did not suffer as much with surgery pain as he did with stomach gas, one of the major side effects with abdominal surgery. Due to his and Laura's setbacks, it was worse than normal with his abdominal open for so long. He did a lot of required walking and going to the bathroom, but neither did any good.

Visiting Doug we could not tell if he was happy or not to see us. Having to endure higher blood sugar levels than normal due to the surgery and medications, he appeared tired and withdrawn – not smiling or talking much. One could see the mood swings, personality change, and depression setting in.

With Dr. Ball's guidance, Doug's diabetes had been in good control for the past two years. But now that he had the surgery, he was completely out of control! Looking at him in the hospital bed brought back old memories of 19-years-ago when he was first diagnosed as a diabetic. Only this time I thought, we had a much greater challenge to meet!

Knowing his body needs more than anyone, Doug knew he was not getting enough insulin his body required at that time, and he was very upset about it. After complaining to the nurses, they informed Doug they would rather have his sugar run a bit higher than lower for fear of insulin reactions.

"My blood sugars runnin' sky high!" he snarled, telling me later what they had told him. Doug was irate knowing his sugar was high. He was feeling it and scared, knowing just what damage it could do. Unsatisfied with the nurses reasoning, he approached the transplant doctors later that day. "If I have to stay in here," he told them, "I want full control of my diabetes! Can I do my sugar tests and give myself shots?" he asked.

Doug got along with all of his doctors, especially Dr. Shaver and Dr. Jonsson. Having found no problem with it, they gave Doug permission to have insulin, needles, and a blood machine. Therefore, Doug was pleased that he could manage his own diabetes for the rest of the time he was in the hospital.

Fear of Going Home: On February 13, five days after surgery, Doug was released from the hospital. To keep check on his Creatinine count for kidney rejection, he was told to return three times a week for the first three months to have his blood checked. But in Doug's case, we found, the trips would be more frequent. During the time of his release, we had no idea what all Doug had yet to go through, nor did he.

At the time of his release, he was still very weak and barely able to walk. Feeling uneasy about leaving, Doug was petrified of coming home. "I just feel more secure and safe here," he had told us, in wanting to stay because he felt so bad. Although the nurse assured him he would be all right, Doug still felt doubtful. Before leaving, he was told to return the next morning for blood work to be done.

Doug had a full-time job just caring for himself when he came home from the hospital. Throughout the day, he would have to measure his weight, the in-put and out-put of fluids, readings on his blood pressure, body temperature, and his blood sugar, as well as keeping time on all the pills he had to take. He was told to keep all information-logged daily in a ledger book that was given to him when he was discharged. Being needed, so the transplant team could review it with each trip back.

Doug also had a major endeavor in itself, just trying to manage his diabetes. With most of his medications causing increased blood sugar levels, he was taking nine to ten insulin shots a day. Not to mention all the finger pricks he had to do, to which he said he felt like a pincushion.

Rejection: When discharged after the transplant, Sharon took Doug back to the hospital the following morning for blood work. Showing a slight increase in his Creatinine count, she had to take him back each day.

Although Doug had been on dialysis, his creatinine count at seven was still considered high at the time of his transplant. After surgery it had dropped into the low ones, but had steadily risen to a 2.8 upon his release. With blood work now showing a count of 3.3 and showing signs of rejection, he was admitted on February 16, just eight days after his initial surgery. An immune response against grafted tissue, which if not successfully treated, would result in failure of the graft to survive.

First Admission: It was snowing lightly that Friday morning on February 16, 1996, only to get heavier as the day wore on. I received a phone call from Sharon at the hospital, saying they were going to keep Doug overnight. Also to let me know if the snow continued, she would be staying over with him. If she did, she wanted to know if I could pick up Melissa from day-care that evening and watch her overnight.

By mid-day, several inches of snow had fallen. With the day-care closing early, Sharon called again, to inform me that her friend's Kevin and Pat, whom also had a daughter in the same class, had offered to bring Melissa home for me. "That way," she said, "you won't have to go out in all this snow to get her."

Melissa being a smart two-and-a-half year old understood where her Mommy and Daddy were that day. Seeing her Daddy on dialysis and the visit at the hospital after his transplant, she knew he had been sick. During his hospital stay, Melissa had trouble sleeping at nights – waking up and crying for her daddy. Sharon would ease her fears by telling her that he was all right, and would be home soon.

Melissa loved her Daddy and missed him dearly during that time, as he had always entertained her in the evenings by running around, and roughhousing with her. She was such a runabout, so full of life

– being so typical of her dad at that age. We had no problem with Melissa staying over that snowy night, but Doug and Sharon did not do as well in the hospital.

Steroids: Having settled in his room, Doug was given massive doses of steroids to prevent transplant rejection, by oral and injection, which caused him to be jittery and feeling what he called, "like climbing the walls." He had also developed severe constipation. It was an effect from all the pills he had to take, and was told if it was not corrected by the next morning, he would be given an enema. They informed him at that time, that he could not go home until he had a bowel movement. Needless to say, this was all Doug had to hear to set him off. So far, he thought he had been through almost everything there was to go through, but taking an enema – he didn't think so!

However, to put it bluntly, he loudly informed, "They are not going to stick anything up my butt!!" Worrying about the enema, as well as being on a steroid high, he did not get much rest by having tossed and turned throughout the night. Paying for the use of a vacant bed next to Doug, Sharon was unable to sleep as well due to all his fretting.

"I kept hearing all these toilets flushing all night," he said, annoyed, the next morning. "I wish it could've been me doin' the flushing," he remarked sighing. With his nurse knowing how upset he would be in having an enema, she gave him a rectal suppository instead. Although he was given a suppository, it really wasn't necessary. What really sent him to the bathroom was hearing that the wind had torn off his storm door. Although, upset about the storm door, he still rejoiced by yelling "Hallelujah" - being thankful he had a bowel movement. Accomplishing this ordeal, he was discharged the next morning on Sunday, February 18, with a Creatinine count of 2.7 down from 3.3 when admitted.

Racing Friend: Shortly after Doug's release from the hospital, I received a phone call from "Skeet" Camden, a former racing friend. She wanted to know how Doug and Laura were doing, and then she told me she thought their transplant should make local news. "Skeet" asked me if it would be all right if she got in touch with someone she knew at Potomac News, our local newspaper.

"I think it would make a great human-interest story," she said.

"I'm sick and tired of reading nothing but bad news all the time," she remarked bitterly.

"I think it's time we have some good news printed for a change, don't you?" she asked.

Doing so, "Skeet" called back to tell me that the Potomac News was very interested in doing an article on Doug and Laura. "They'll be getting in touch with you soon," she said.

Not realizing it would be so soon, I was contacted the next day. Wanting to set up an appointment, I informed Larsia, the reporter, that Doug was not doing too well. I told her that he had just been released from the hospital, and that I would get in touch with him to find out if he was up to having an interview at that time.

Self-Conscious: In additional to all the steroids that had been previously injected, Doug was taking, orally, 60 milligrams of Prednisone daily. Prednisone, a synthetic cortisone-like steroid routinely used to reduce inflammation, is also given with other medications to prevent transplant rejection. Its immunosuppressant effect is attributed to a reduced production of lymphocytes and antibodies. It carries several side effects, with two of them, fluid retention and acne.

Due to the effects from all the medications and the Prednisone Doug was taking, changed his facial features somewhat. Causing rounding of the face ("moon face") as they call it from the Prednisone, his face appeared swollen and puffy. And though he did not have "bad acne," he did have a few blemishes, which he became very self-conscious of. Having a flawless complexion, he would literally go to pieces whenever he would get any type of blemish on his face. As in the past, he had always doted on himself to a certain extent. At times, he would tease by flexing his muscles – pretending he was a somewhat macho-man.

Not feeling well and thinking his appearance was not up to par when Larisa called, he was not all that excited about having an interview. Having had his transplant two weeks prior and just being discharged from an additional three-day stay, he did not feel up to an interview, let on, having his picture taken too. However, he insisted, if Laura was up to it, then he would be too. With Laura and Doug's approval, I set up an appointment with Larisa for the following week, February 26.

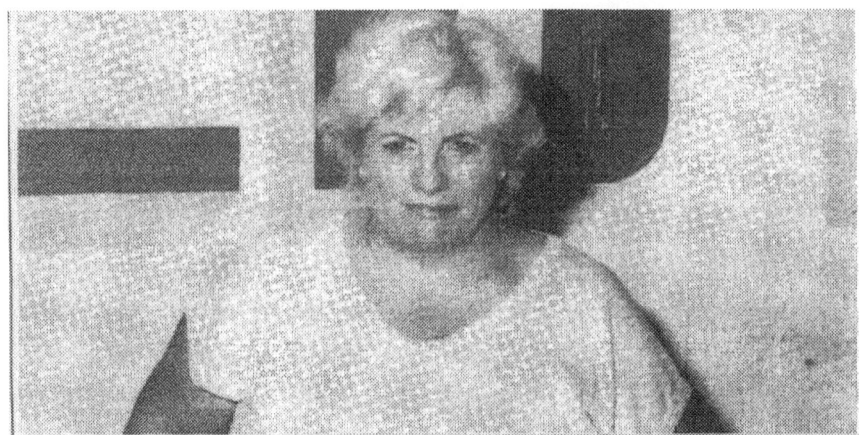

Juanita (Skeet) Camden, a former racing friend, that drove the #41, white and blue Pinto in the Mini Stock Division, made the connection to have transplant article published in our local newspaper.

CHAPTER 15

OKT3 TREATMENT * BIOPSY * SELLING MODIFIED

Second admission: Doug continued his trips to the hospital for follow up blood work. In eight-days time his creatinine went from 3.3 to 3.5. Still showing signs of rejection after his transplant 18-days prior, he was readmitted on Monday, February 26, the same day as our scheduled interview with Larisa. Not knowing in advance that he was going to be admitted, I immediately called her from the hospital and gave her all the details. Having to postpone our afternoon interview, I rescheduled at a later date.

When admitted, Doug was introduced to a new treatment – a drug called OKT3. We were told that this drug was used for being more specific, for cells that could cause rejection. It is given intravenously, with side effects that include increased susceptibility to infections, fevers, shortness of breath (particularly with the first treatment), joint pains, swelling, hepatitis and kidney dysfunction. Doug was told the OKT3 would be given to him on an outpatient basis after the first few treatments.

He was given his first treatment around 8:00 that night. When leaving him earlier that evening, I can still recall how sad and depressed he looked. With arms crossed over his stomach and eyes closed, one could almost feel, and comprehend, the conflicting torment his body and mind was going through. Before leaving, we were told he would be watched very closely throughout the night for any bad side effects.

Returning the next day, we found him not looking nor feeling very well. "Every joint in my body aches," he weakly informed. "Just like I had the flu. I ran a temperature last night," he said, sniffling. "I did a lot of sweating too, but I didn't have any trouble breathing like they thought I would." Then he told us that Doctor Jonsson and Doctor Shaver stayed until he had his injection. "They wanted to make sure I was going to be all right before going home. They even came in to see me before leaving," he boasted, elated they were that concerned about him.

Ultra-Sound & Biopsy Test: During this crucial period, Dr. Shaver would perform yet another kidney biopsy on Doug's kidney, as well as requesting an ultrasound test. Ultrasound is used to produce pictures of structures within the body by sound waves of extremely high frequency (more than 20,000 vibrations per second. Done by a controlled beam that is directed into the body where the echoes of reflected sound is used to form an electronic image. With the advantages that the patient is not submitted to potentially harmful radiation and that structures not opaque to X-rays can be seen.

Having revealed a formation of peritransplant fluid collection with the ultrasound, it was drained successfully under ultrasound guidance. Doug's skin was anesthetized first, whereupon, a large suction type needle was inserted through the abdominal area, withdrawing fluid on three different intervals.

"They got a lot of fluid off," Doug told us after the procedure. "The fluid was a pale yellow and it had all these little particles floating around in it," he continued, giving us details while squinting his eyes in disgust.

After having had the ultrasound, Dr. Shaver performed the kidney biopsy in Doug's hospital room. As I turned to leave, Dr. Shaver smiled and told me, "You don't have to leave. You can stay and watch." Hesitant to see the process done, I kept my distance by viewing very little from across the room.

Dr. Shaver started the procedure by numbing Doug's stomach. He then made a small nick in the skin with a knife, whereupon, the automated biopsy needle was introduced through the skin into the kidney itself. The biopsy gun was fired and a core of kidney tissue was obtained. Two additional passes were made in a similar fashion. Showing Doug and I a small sliver of kidney tissue that he'd taken, Dr. Shaver informed that it would be sent to the lab to be analyzed.

An Ordeal: Doug did not mind having the biopsy, but was not thrilled by having to remain calm, and flat on his back for four long hours. This was a prevention that required a five-pound sandbag applied over the bandage site to prevent any further bleeding in the kidney area.

This was not the first time Doug had to go through this, as other tests he had taken required the same technique. It reminded me of what we went through one day in this position, when he was due his medication. What an ordeal it was for him, and for me, as I tried to elevate his head high enough while he took twenty-some pills.

"They still feel like they're stuck in my throat," he complained, taking five or six at a time with very little water.

"Take one at a time," I told him, with some of them being large pills and not able to drink a lot in one given time.

"It'll take me forever if I did that," he snapped back as he held his hand out for a few more.

"Try to drink more water then!"

"They still feel like they're stuck," he'd say, after having drank more. I could fully understand what he was going through as it gagged me just watching. Having achieved this, he started belching and complaining that he didn't feel well.

It is devastating to see your child have to suffer – no matter what age they are. If he wasn't a diabetic, I thought, all this would be so much easier on him. Then realizing, if he wasn't a diabetic, he wouldn't be going through any of this at all! They say the Lord does not put more on you than you can bear, but the trying times we've had, I felt, we were certainly being tested.

Weekly Treatment: With all tests completed, and having had five OKT3 treatments within five days, Doug was discharged from the

115

hospital on March 1. Coming home with a 2.7 creatinine count, down from 3.5 when he was admitted. With his biopsy test showing he had a mild cellular rejection, his doctors were hoping the OKT3 treatments would take care of it. Normally, one has a ten-day treatment with the OKT3, whereas, Doug had to endure twelve. With Sharon back to work, I took him to the hospital each morning for his remaining treatments, with Sharon taking him on the weekend when she was off.

During one of our weekly morning trips, Doug became very sick. I barely got the car parked when he vomited. "I hope no one saw me do this," he said shyly, as he cleaned up the mishap he made in the hospital parking lot. He said that drinking a diet sprite on the way, mixed with pills he had taken earlier, did not agree with his stomach.

Weak and pale looking, Doug walked slowly as we made our way toward the hospital. When entering the treatment room on the eighth floor, the space was small. There, he was connected intravenously for his treatment, which took approximately forty-five minutes to an hour. The attending nurse had a difficult time getting the IV in, as Doug dreaded the IV more so than the treatment itself. "I don't know why they always do," he would say afterward. "They never seem to have any trouble down in the lab!" he voiced bitterly.

While Doug and I waited for his turn that day, we encountered a young man whom looked to be in his twenties. Having lost all of his hair, we figured he was there for some type of cancer treatment. Making conversation with him, we could almost visualize what a horrible ordeal he and his family were going through.

"He's been talking a lot lately," his mother whispered to me, as her son chatted on while rubbing his legs. "I guess they'll be all right," he muttered, being optimistic to why his legs were hurting so bad. Leaving that day, Doug realized he was not the only one suffering and having to cope with a lot of misfortunes in his lifetime. "I sure feel sorry for that guy," he said sadly. "You think you have it bad until you see someone like that." Confronted with this, Doug kept a better outlook on things for a while.

Selling Modified: Shortly after his release from the hospital in early March, Doug sold his modified. With race season drawing near and knowing he would never be able to race again, he could no longer look at his ready-to-go race car that sat under our garage carport. It brought back too many memories, as it was something he could no longer do – just as in the past. As well as knowing he had made a promise to his sister, which he intended to keep.

Although he knew what he had to do, it still did not make him that happy. Not feeling well to begin with and having to sell his race car was complete torment for him. I watched from the kitchen window, that cool March day, as he went back and forth gathering parts, tires, and all the accessories that went with the race car. With mouth gripped firmly, his expression revealed nothing but sadness and bitterness with each trip he made. It was like watching a part of his life go by. Other than Sharon and Melissa, racing was the next meaningful thing in his life. I could sense the heartbreak he was now going through.

As the new owner pulled away with the race car, Doug's only comment to us was, "We need the money!" With all the expense they had with doctors, buying a house, as well as having volunteered to pay Laura for the seven weeks she had to take leave after surgery, had put them in a financial bind. Although Laura's job found no fault to give her the time off, they were not obligated to pay. "It's the least I can do for her," Doug had said, in giving him one of her kidneys.

Although Doug had finally received his first disability check along with all back pay the day before his transplant surgery, it did not take long to go by having paid bills. Having filed for disability nearly two years prior, it was given to him only by having been on Dialysis, which automatically qualifies one for disability.

Thirty-Third Birthday: Shortly after selling his race car, Doug celebrated his 33rd birthday on March 20 with his family. As in the past, I prepared his favorite dinner, lasagna, and baked his favorite cake – yellow with chocolate frosting. With his transplant just six weeks prior, and to all he had been through, we tried lifting his spirits some, though, we could have used some too.

Third Admission: Not doing any better, and with further signs of rejection, Doug was admitted to the hospital four days after his birthday. Retaining fluid due to a decrease in urination, his ankles had tripled in size and his creatinine had jumped back to 3.3. Not only was he given, at that time, massive doses of lasix, a diuretic, orally and by injection to take the fluid off, but he was also given massive doses of steroids again. The steroids making his body, he says, feeling unattached.

It was found that the same formation of fluid that was drained successfully by ultrasound nearly a month ago had reaccumulated. Whereupon, laparoscopic surgery was scheduled – a procedure done by a viewing tube that is inserted through the abdominal wall. Performed by his doctor the next day, a temporary tube was inserted for drainage, placed, within a small opening that was made on the outer abdominal. Doug was discharged from the hospital two days later.

Doug was happy to return home with ankles reduced to a normal size and a creatinine count down to 2.5 from 3.3 when admitted. Due to the procedure though, and what all he had been through in the past, he was feeling very tired and worn down. So much so, that he was beginning to dislike his home away from home – the seventh floor at Fairfax Hospital.

Interview: Being persistent in wanting to set up an appointment for our interview, Larisa, from Potomac News kept calling several times during the month of March. With all of Doug's setbacks, we never found the time before. It always seemed when it was a good time for her it never was for us, or vice-versa. Giving Doug a few days rest after his release from the hospital, I called Larisa, finally setting a time for the next day.

Larisa met us at Doug and Sharon's late that afternoon, bringing Rhonda, the photographer with her. The interview went well with

Rhonda taking several photo shots of Doug and Laura, as well as Doug and Melissa. When leaving, we were told the article would be published soon, and that we would be notified a few days prior to its release.

CHAPTER 16

URETERAL STENT * EXPLORATORY SURGERY

Fourth Admission: Shortly after the interview, Doug was admitted to the hospital on April 19 for the removal of a ureteral stent. Doctor Hardy, Laura's urologist, surgically inserted it at the time of the transplant. Required for kidney transplant patients, the stent is placed at the time of surgery to help aid healing of an anastomosis (the surgical suturing of blood vessels), by draining the contents away. Because of the healing process, a stent is not removed for a certain amount of time after surgery, but Doug's remained three weeks longer than he was told it would be.

I stayed by Doug's bedside that morning while we waited for them to take him away for the procedure. Doug's only concern at that time was wanting to know if he was going to be given any type of anesthesia. He had enough pain, and he wanted to be put out. Doctor Shaver eased his mind before taking him, saying that he would probably be given something.

Returning after the procedure, Doug was irate. "They didn't give me anything!" he groaned, while giving me the details of what he had gone through and how much it had hurt. "My whole rear-end came off the table when Dr. Hardy took it out," he squawked, in having to take the stent out through his penis. "He wanted to know if I wanted to look at the stent?" I told him, "Hell No!"

Doug continued to be irate by having the added worry of his blood sugar, since he was not allowed any food past midnight the night before. "I could've eaten this morning if I knew they weren't going to put me out," he griped. He survived the ordeal, but wondered what he would encounter next – it did not take long...

Fifth Admission: Just eleven days after having the stent removed, Doug was admitted on April 30 with complaints of a bloated feeling through the abdominal area, plus, a decrease in urine output again. His symptoms of pressure to the kidney and bladder led the doctors to believe they were dealing with a fluid condition. They gave him an ultrasound, which confirmed this, and was told he had to undergo exploratory surgery, for what they now call "the fluid," a recurrent peritransplant lymphocele. Discharged the next day, he was told to return in eight days for surgery.

Sixth Admission: Admitted for the sixth time since his February transplant, Doug underwent exploratory surgery on May 8 under Dr. Shaver's guidance, with Doctors Jonsson, and Roslynn Mason as his assistants. After adequate general anesthesia was obtained, an incision was made through the skin in the line where the previous incision was used for the renal transplant, in the left lower section of the abdomen.

In the operative findings, there was a large fluid collection found near the kidney, as well as the ureter - the tube leading from the kidney to the bladder to which the fluid was drained. However, due to more fluid found than expected, two additional openings were made in the abdominal to foresee where it was being originated. The doctors finding what they thought was causing the problem, they completed the surgery by placing a single drain overlying the ureter for drainage.

After incisions were stitched and sterile dressings were applied, Doug was taken to the recovery room and listed in stable condition. Tolerating the surgery well, he was discharged three days later on May 11.

A kidney biopsy during this period, revealed a small mass of chronic inflammatory cells adjacent to the tubules of the kidneys. Doug's biopsy was diagnosed as: Mild acute cellular rejection.

Seventh Admission: Fifteen days later on May 26, he was admitted to the hospital for the same scenario. A decrease in urination, as well as his creatinine count going up to 6.9 - the highest it had been since the transplant.

On admission, he underwent an ultrasound that revealed a lymphocele on the lower section of the kidney, which an output of 80cc of fluid was drained under ultrasound guidance. Also, a catheter was placed for drainage after finding a collection toward the back of the kidney that could not be drained under ultrasound.

Kidney Cut: During the process of injecting the catheter tube, which was viewed on his own and not by machine guidance, the ultrasound-attending physician accidentally nicked Doug's kidney. "Oops!" the physician said, "Did you feel that?" Although Doug had, he did not say much – only later...

With the kidney being cut, the ultrasound physician did not want to take the catheter tube out for fear of internal bleeding. To prevent this from happening, it was taped and left in place. Whereupon, the physician had to make an additional opening beneath that one, so another catheter could be placed for drainage. This was the fifth opening in his abdomen in fifteen days.

It was bad enough having the kidney cut, let alone having to go through what he dreaded the most – lying on his back with the five-pound sandbag placed on his abdomen for four long hours again. By the time Doug arrived to his room, he was steaming. "I know accidents happen, but why me?" he grumbled. "My poor kidney. I sure didn't need this to happen. I'm having enough problems as it is. He should have used the machine to find my kidney instead of guessing where it was!" he continued, extremely upset over the whole ordeal.

Doug was disappointed too, knowing due to the freak incident he had to stay in the hospital longer than planned. "If they hadn't cut my kidney," he voiced angrily, in having to stay for fear of it bleeding, "I would've been out of here today!" On the fifth day, Doug anxiously waited for the catheter that nicked his kidney to be removed. The second one underneath would be left for drainage. Not removing the catheter until late that evening, Dr. Jonsson released him around 7:30 p.m. on May 31. His creatinine fell from 6.9 to 2.8, and was urinating without difficulty upon discharge. He was given instructions to follow-up in the transplant center.

Trying to Find a Solution: Doug's fluid condition had all the doctors at the transplant center baffled. Doctors Jonsson and Shaver had told us they had never witnessed a case such as his. Upset to what all Doug had been through, and thinking his condition might have been encountered elsewhere, they had called other transplant hospitals trying to find a solution.

Unfortunately, there was not a case to be found like his. "I'd have to be the odd ball," Doug said, when hearing. "We're not giving up," they told him. Doug had faith in Doctor Jonsson and Shaver; in fact, they had seen each other so frequently they were like long, lost friends.

Doug made a lot of friends at the hospital during the time he had been there. The doctors, nurses, and receptionist thought a lot of him. Starting from the tenth floor transplant center all the way to the lab on the basement floor. It was easy to understand why, the past four months he had practically lived there. In fact, so much so that he mentioned about renting an apartment close by, claiming, that it would save him time traveling to and from.

Eighth Admission: Doug's traveling did not get better with time. Discharged just four days prior, he came down with a flu-bug and was readmitted on June 4. He was vomiting and had diarrhea, so Doug was given an IV for dehydration and was told if all went well he could go home the next day.

However, still showing signs of rejection, Doctors Jonsson and Shaver told Doug he would be given a new treatment called Sclerotherapy, telling him, that it would be given to him before he was released.

CHAPTER 17

SCLEROTHERAPY TREATMENT
*
SURGERY (BIG ONE)
*
TORNADO

Burning Pain: Sclerotherapy is a treatment used by injecting an irritant solution into a vein in order to clot it, and to get fibrous tissue to form within it. It is mainly used to treat varicose veins. The doctors were in hopes that this treatment would help clot the lymphatic (fluid) condition that Doug suffered through so much with.

Feeling better the next day, and before treatment, he was premedicated with five mg of Valium and five mg of Morphine by IV. The irritant solution consisted of a mixture of five hundred milligrams of Doxycycline, an antibiotic, and 30cc of normal saline, which they injected into the kidney area through the drainage catheter into his abdomen.

I was going to get Doug after he was released that day, but was told not to come until I heard from him first. I received the call right after they had injected him. When answering, I could tell by the tone of his voice that he was in a lot of pain. "My whole stomach feels like it's on fire," he uttered weakly. "It's just a constant burning feeling, like somebody put a hot blowtorch in my stomach. It hurt so bad my whole body shook," he said. Then he told me he did not know if he could go

127

through it again. Doug did not know how many treatments he would have, but knew it would depend on how well he responded to them. Released that day in late afternoon on June 5, he was told to come back in five days for his second treatment. It would be sooner...

Treatment At Home: Developing an oozing leak in one of the openings near his navel site due to surgery ten days prior, he had to return the next day for an extra stitch. Doug returned to the hospital on June 10 and 13 for repeated sclerotherapy treatment, but he was released on his own to administer his own treatment every morning at home.

Doug would dispense the premixed solution into his kidney through the catheter, which was connected to a plastic bag that was attached to his left leg. The same tube that dispensed it, also disposed of it. The disposed fluid was reddish-brown in color and carried a lot of what he says, "nasty looking debris." Clogging the tube periodically, Doug would have to syringe and clean out the catheter. He would sit straddled-legged on the commode to accomplish this ordeal by dropping its contents in water. He used this treatment at home for five days, at which time, he still complained of lower abdominal pain.

Fluid that continued to recur around the transplanted kidney despite multiple drainage attempts, including laparoscopic surgery, and Doug showing no improvement during this period, Doctor Shaver readmitted him.

Ninth Admission: On June 24, 1996, Doug walked wearily as he entered Fairfax Hospital, knowing, he would be undergoing a second exploratory surgery - with this one being marked on our calendar as the "Big One." He was not aware of the extent of his surgery prior to going in, other than the doctors saying they were determined to find the reason for all his setbacks.

This surgery would be much greater than in the past, as there would not be any small openings made this time. Doctor Shaver, being assisted by Jonsson and Mason, would begin their task – to find the actual cause of Doug's pre-existing fluid problem in efforts to rid him of the, so called, lymphocele that plagued him.

After Doug was prepped and draped in a sterile fashion and given anesthesia, a midline incision was made from the navel all the way to the bottom of the abdomen. Once opened, the colon was carefully freed from its lateral attachments so that the membrane overlying the kidney could be visualized. A lot of purulent (pus) material was suctioned and flushed from this cavity and sent for culture. It was found that this cavity; however, was not the same cavity that was previously being drained by the percutaneous catheter prior to surgery, which the drainage fluid was then clear.

Having freed the kidney from its attachment, it was noted that the kidney and the inguinal (groin) ligament were extremely tight against the outside abdominal wall. This began causing pockets to form, which led the doctors to believe this may have made it difficult to previously drain the lymphoceles. They thought healing too fast in an abnormal way, caused it. Normally the body heals from the inside out, whereas, it looked as if Doug had healed from the outside in.

With the surgery over and bleeding assured, a Reliavac drain was placed through the right lower abdominal wall and into the previously drained abscess cavity. Doug was then taken to the recovery room in stable condition, without any noted complications.

Tornado: While Vic, Sharon and I waited that afternoon in the lobby for Doug to return to his room from surgery, there was a violent storm brewing outside that we were not aware of. Being thirsty, I went to the transplant unit on the tenth floor to get a soda. As I neared the vending machine at the end of the hall, I saw nothing but pure darkness through the large glass-plated window. Even with it being mid-afternoon, it looked as if it were night out. My heart raced as I watched the dark-covered clouds hover lowly in the greenish-black sky. Gazing down upon the street, as I got closer to the window, I could see the treetops bending and swaying from the high winds. I have to hurry, I thought, as I got my soda. Racing back to the elevator, I was anxious to get off the top floor.

Arriving on the seventh floor, Vic and Sharon were waiting for me. Telling them about the storm, we went into Doug's hospital room to further pursue the weather condition. Standing at the large picture window, I heard a distant roar - like a train sound.

"Listen," I said, "Do you hear that?"

"Hear what?" Vic answered, as he and Sharon came closer to the window.

"That roaring sound," I repeated.

"Just like Dorothy in the Wizard of Oz! Huh?" Sharon says, with me thinking the sound might be a tornado.

"That's just the roar of the air conditioners," Vic adds, laughing, with both of them thinking I was just hearing things. I could understand their reasoning; after all, our immediate area was not known for its tornados. It seldom happened. However, to be on the safe side, we each went back to the hallway to stay clear of the large glass plated window.

It was comforting to know Doug's surgery was over with in case the electricity went out. Vic reminded me that the hospital would have had generators as a back up if it had. Shortly thereafter, we returned to Doug's room. "Maybe we can get some news on the weather," Sharon said, as she turned on the TV. "Who knows, we may have had a tornado!" she joked, still making fun of my hearing a roaring sound. Rain was beating hard against the windowpane, making it difficult to see out when we heard the announcement.

"A tornado touched down south-east of Interstate 495 in Fairfax," the newscaster announced. "I told you I heard a roaring sound!" I exclaimed, with the tornado touching down just a few miles from the hospital. "You were right!" Sharon said, totally surprised. "And here we made fun of you," she said, apologizing. Knowing there were no casualties since the tornado was small, we were thankful.

"Big" Incision: Doug was brought back to his room that day in late afternoon. Seeing him attached to tubes, IV, catheters and such, was becoming an all too familiar sight. Heavily sedated from surgery, he was alert enough to inform us that he had the "big" incision.

"They cut me all the way down this time," he muttered softly, with a groan.

"They gave you a C-Section," I teased.

"A what?"

"A women's C-Section," I repeated, smiling.

"You know? When you have a baby!"

"Oh," he replied, expressionless. We told him about the tornado, but I don't think anything we said registered with him. With his eyes closed, he fell back into a sedated sleep.

On the way home that night, we were amazed by all the trees that had fallen by the roadside on Interstate 495. The damage from the storm, I thought on the drive home, was mild compared to what Doug's mind, body and soul had been put through in the past few years. With the following days to come being no better, he would be going through trying times – ones, he longs to forget....

Recovery: After Doug's "big" surgery, as what he called it, he was placed on Vancomycin, an antibacterial antibiotic, due to abscess fluid found at the time of surgery. Later he was put on Bactrim by IV for two days, but then switched back to Vancomycin in finding that it did better. Because of the abscess, Dr. Mary Schmidt, the infectious disease doctor, would keep check on Doug with the transplant team. Also, having had a kidney biopsy at the time of surgery that showed moderate acute cellular rejection that had increased from his last surgery, Doug was started on Solu Medrol – a Cortison drug to control the reduction.

Losing Patience: Doug's hospital stay was not pleasant. Having to encounter several bothersome situations, along with others he had to deal with, left him highly agitated. To prevent any gas pressure that might cause further discomfort to his already mangled insides, he was placed on a liquid diet. Hungry for solid food, he dreaded when mealtime came.

The day after surgery, they had him up walking. He cringed at the thought of that too. It was difficult enough for him to sit up in bed, let alone get out of it. When he did manage, he would place one hand on the IV pole for support, while using the other to hold his hospital gown together in the back. And with a urethral catheter dangling between his legs, he would slowly pace on. It was a sight to see him walk, as he looked comical and pitiful all at the same time. Not knowing by watching him, if one should laugh or cry. Doug continued this routine several times a day. So much that he got tired of holding his gown together in the back, and just said, "The hell with it! If they wanna look at my butt then let'em look." And that he did – he just did not care anymore.

Hygiene Conscious: On the third day of his hospital stay, I received an early morning phone call from him.

"Mom" he said, "When you come today, can you bring some shampoo and help me wash my hair? It's so oily I can't stand it! They gave me some dry shampoo, but it doesn't work that well."

"I hate to bother you," he said, concerned, "but I can't bend over that far to wash it on my own."

"I'll be glad when I can take a shower too," he continued, in not being able because of the IV and catheters. Hygiene conscious, he was upset over his hair and not able to bathe. By the time I arrived that afternoon, Doug was an unhappy champ. Being temperamental, he was moody, sensitive, and touchy. Lord knows he had reason to be, his body had been put through a lot in the past few days. It had been cut, probed, and jabbed on – inside and out. His abdomen had so many scars, that Doug had previously commented that his stomach was beginning to look like a road map.

I waited for Doug to get out of bed, in which he had to position himself several different ways to maneuver him-self out. Not able to stand straight, he walked slowly, hunched over to the bathroom. By the time we got there, I could see his jaw tighten. "Just look at this!" he yelled, watching blood drip down his stomach onto the floor. "This is ridiculous," he fumed. Frustrated, with plans to remove it in a few days, the catheter tube was inserted within the abdomen without stitching.

Trying to prevent further bleeding from the loosely hung catheter while washing his hair, Doug stood, leaning, with hands outstretched on the bathroom sink. Surrounded by dangling tubes, an IV pole and such, it was hard knowing what position he or I should get into, to master this great task. "I sure feel better," he commented, after I finished, which lifted his spirits some. "Thanks Mom!" he told me.

His good mood didn't last though, by the time Sharon arrived that evening, she didn't find him as pleasant. In part by not feeling well, and upset to what all he had been through.

Bad Attitude: Although he had not eaten much and did a lot of walking, he still suffered gas discomfort due to the surgery. Making matters worse, his blood sugar was running wacky again, which did not help his attitude any. He was given additional steroid treatment that did not help either, as on the fourth day he went off on his doctors. Having had a bad day, his eyes glared as his temper burst forth. "Are you going to fix this kidney or not? If not, then take the damn thing out!" he raged.

The doctors promised him they would find the problem, and although they thought they had fixed it, only time would tell. In the meantime, Doug's patience was running thin. He was hurting in more ways than one and the doctors knew it. They fully understood the frustration he was going through. "If the doctors told me I had just a week to live," he later remarked, "I wouldn't have cared. That's just how bad I felt." During this period it was more than he could withstand. His life was in turmoil to which he saw no way out.

Although Doug didn't want us coming to see him everyday for fear of it being too much on us, I still went during the afternoon hours and Sharon went after work in the evenings. We wondered if he wanted us there at all. As much as he missed Melissa, he did not want Sharon to bring her to see him. Looking as bad as he felt, he did not want her seeing him that way. Melissa worried about her daddy and he did not want that. Although Sharon took her once, it didn't seem to upset her – she knew her daddy had been sick. Just being able to see him made her feel better. She'd missed him.

Catheter Removed: Doug not only had a drain catheter placed within the surgery site, but also one within the kidney too. Prior to going home, Dr. Jonsson took two syringes of fluid from the catheter that was placed within Doug's kidney. He was told that the tubes would be taken out completely before going home that day.

Later that afternoon, an assistant doctor came to Doug's room. Knowing he would be able to go home once it was done, the first thing Doug asked, was, "When will the catheters be taken out?" "Now!" the doctor replied.

"Take a big breath and hold it," the doctor told him as he began pulling ten inches of ball like tubing from the kidney and surgery site. "I can still hear the sound of it," Doug recalled taking the tubes out. "It was a flapping sound – like chilled Jell-0 being poured. It was weird sounding!" he said, squinting his face.

Drive Home: Released on the sixth day, he came home late that afternoon on June 29. Working that Saturday, as engineer, for Shenandoah Pride Dairy and just minutes from the hospital, his dad went and got him. Caught in a traffic jam on Interstate I-95 on a hot-humid day just prolonged Doug's misery. Not helping him any, by having to turn off the air conditioner in his dad's 1972 Chevy Blazer, for fear it would over-heat.

Feeling sick because of the heat, Doug barely made it out of the blazer before vomiting in the driveway when they arrived home. "I held it as long as I could," he told us, while hosing the driveway. Then he told us why he had gotten sick. Doug said his lunch had been brought to him just prior to leaving. "Anxious to leave", he said, "I just grabbed a banana from the food tray to eat on the way home." Although he knew his blood sugar was low at the time, he thought the banana would hold him over, with him not knowing, the trip from the hospital would take so long. "Between the heat, low blood sugar and eating an over-ripped banana," he said, "Is what did me in."

Fourth of July: In a week's time, Doug seemed to be doing better. With the holiday coming, he was looking forward to our annual Fourth of July get together. As in the past, all our friends and families would gather each year at Isaac Walton, the same Lodge where Doug and

Sharon were married. As each family brought meat, main dish and dessert, we always ended up with an over-abundance of food.

Our outings were not only known for their good food, but also for our yearly annual horseshoe tournaments. Volleyball and softball games would be played too, as well as games and prizes for all the little ones. Some would even bring fishing poles so they could go fishing in the nearby pond.

Considering what all Doug had previously been through, everyone thought he looked well. Although he could not join any of the activities, he did enjoy watching all others, as well as all the good food.

Tenth Admission: Doug had to go back to the hospital the next day on July 5 for additional blood work. Showing an increased creatinine count, he was admitted that day to undergo Sclerotherapy again. The catheter tube that was removed from his kidney site just six days prior would have to be placed back in.

The following morning on the sixth, Doug was premedicated with 5mg of Valium orally, and 5mg of Morphine by IV – just as before. As the irritant solution entered into his already irritated kidney cavity, he developed severe pain. More so than before, that he had to be redosed with an additional 3 mg of IV Morphine.

With the severity of it all, the catheter was left within the kidney with the bag attached to his left leg when he was released that day. When will it end? I thought, with him having to do this all over again. I just did not know how much more his body could take – nor did he.

Eleventh Admission: Doug returned to the hospital three days later on July 9 for repeated blood work. Finding that his creatinine had gone from 2.7 to 2.9 in spite of the Scleotherapy treatment, the doctors readmitted him. That day, a kidney biopsy was performed to evaluate for rejection, and possible OKT3 – antilymphocyte therapy again.

With the biopsy still showing acute moderate rejection, it was felt that this was probably the cause of his Chronic Lymph production – the fluid that is derived from connective tissues and tissues between organs. Doug was informed at that time, he would have to repeat the OKT3 treatment – a serum containing antibodies that surpress lymphocytic activity. Doug knew what he had to look forward to. He had been through it all before. When told, his shoulders slumped. Only showing emotions through sadden, misty eyes.

Late that afternoon, he was given his first OKT3 treatment by IV injection. This time, he ran a low-grade fever and was nauseous. As before, the doctors kept close watch on him. On the second day, he was given separate, double treatment. In the morning he was given Scleratherapy treatment through his abdomen, and in the afternoon he was given the OKT3 by IV. At which time, his lymphocyte count went from a total of 23 to a total of 2. Three days later on July 11, his creatinine had dropped to just 2.6 – down from 2.9 when he was admitted. With his urine output good, he was discharged that day. He would have fourteen treatments in all, with the first three given while he was in the hospital. The remainder would be given as an outpatient, just as before.

I Can Do It: Doug drove himself back to the hospital each day for his treatment. "You don't have to take me," he would say, by not wanting to take up anymore of my time. "You've done enough already." This would not be the first time he ever went on his own, as he made several trips by himself for blood work, plus, a couple of times when he had to be admitted. He had done it so much that he was getting use to it. "I can do it on my own," he would say.

Going back for his seventh OKT3 treatment on July 15, Dr. Jonsson removed the bag that was connected to Doug's leg. Still having drainage with the bag containing 30cc of fluid, Dr. Jonsson did not remove the catheter, but sealed it with a clear plastic cap in case it had to be used again. Going back to the hospital two days later, 30 more cc's of fluid were suctioned from the catheter prior to his OKT3 treatment. Two days after having his eleventh and final treatment (three less than originally stated) and still having drainage, he was sent home on July 19 with a bag attached to his leg once again.

With Doug's creatinine dropping to 2.1 the doctors felt the treatment did its job, even though fluid was still being discharged. In fact, they had informed Doug, that they doubted his creatinine would get any better. "We'll be pleased if it stays in the low two's," they told him. For all he had been through, it seemed Doug's creatinine count would not get any better. Thinking back, was it all done in vain?

CHAPTER 18

LOSING HOPE
*
LAURA'S INVITATION
*
FRONT PAGE HEADLINE

Losing Weight: Stemming from his last "big" surgery and all the recent treatments he'd been given, by late July, Doug's body was beginning to show all the wear and tear that had been inflicted upon him. Having lost 33 pounds in less than a month, Doug at 6-foot 2-inches tall had gone from 192 pounds down to 159. He was not only looking ill at this time, but he was ill. His once muscle-toned arms were now thin and bony, and there again, dark circles shadowed his sunken eyes.

We worried about him, as well as the doctors. The doctors told him they would have to put him back in the hospital if he did not start eating and putting some weight back on. Informing him that they would give him a couple of weeks before they had to do something about it. "You've got to eat more," they told him, concerned.

Crazy Talk: During this time, he also became very depressed. Being despaired, he was losing hope and giving up. With his demeanor no better as time went on, he began crazy talk. "I ought'a put'a gun to my head," he would say on one of his bad days. Whereupon, demonstrating by pointing a finger to his head. "Oh...Doug. Don't say things like that," I would tell him. It bothered me to hear such talk, but I knew it was coming from being more upset than being serious. His life meant more than that as I had heard him warn time after time, if it wasn't for Melissa! She was his life, he cherished the ground she walked on. Deep down, I knew his irrational thinking at that time was just an impending release from all he had been through. I worried more about him being so poorly in body and spirit then, than in mind.

Stool Test: One week after having had his last OKT3 treatment, the catheter tube and bag were removed from Doug's abdomen on July 26. He was sent home to begin a slow, lingering recovery process. Now that the fluid was controlled, he developed yet another problem – diarrhea. "I'm sure it's one of your medicines causing it." I told him. When Doug confronted the doctors about this, he was told that in order to find the actual cause, they wanted him to have a stool test. A test done by taking stool samples that he would conduct on his own over a three day period. "This is ridiculous!" he said about having to do this. "Who wants to dig around in their own poop?"

Although he thought all of this was absurd – being the typical Doug, he had the receptionists at the doctor's office laughing to what he thought of it all. Within four days after having it done, he received word that his test came back positive. However, this did not help any as he continued having diarrhea, not knowing the cause.

Rebound: Usually after a transplant, it normally takes three months to recover. "You might know I'd be the one," Doug said, with his taking six – twice as long. "That's just my luck." As time went on, his trips to the hospital became less and less. He was beginning to see light at the end of the tunnel. He boasted, that he had broken a record by going a whole week without having to go, or being admitted to the hospital. Still fearful, though, that the fluid might reappear, he kept close watch on his ankles for any signs of swelling. By September, his creatinine had stabilized to 1.9, with him saying he was beginning to feel a lot better. Although his eating habits had picked up some, his weight stayed the same.

Laura's Award: In late September 1996, Laura received an invitation from our then, Governor of Virginia, George Allen. With it stating she was being honored to accept "The Medal of Life" award that would be held at the Marriott Hotel in Richmond, Virginia on November nineteenth. It said that this "special" award was to be given to all living transplant donors, and families from cadaver (deceased) donors. To honor our "hero" with such great praise, with family invited - thirteen of us went.

Our entire family stood applauding when Laura's name was announced that afternoon for her to accept the award from Governor Allen. With the first lady standing next to her husband, the Governor, she smiled and looked at Laura and said, "You're getting a standing ovation!" "Oh, that's just my family!" Laura timidity replied, being shy. Laura had her picture taken that day with the Governor and first lady - proudly displaying her award before her. After the ceremony, our entire clan had pictures taken with them - making it a proud and exciting day.

Donor Donation: Our hearts were with those, though, that accepted the award for their loved (deceased) ones. Sad for their loss, they proudly accepted the award by being honored, in knowing, that their unselfishness and kindness by wanting to help others had helped to save many lives. Their loved ones, like the living donors – giving the "Gift of Life."

The simple fact is that not enough people donate organs. For every 63 people who receive an organ transplant each day nationwide, 17 people die that same day...waiting for the gift of life that did not come in time. And as each year goes by the numbers keep going up.

The National Kidney Foundation of the National Capital Area distributed some disturbing facts. Saying the death rate from kidney disease has been increasing by more than 4.5% each year. In this year of 2005, some 400,000 men, women and children rely on dialysis treatments. Nearly 2,000 new patients are being diagnosed with kidney failure each week, with 90,000 on the waiting list for a transplant. One person can save or enhance the lives of 50 people via organ donation, yet many Americans have never discussed it with their loved ones.

Just by making your wishes known to your family, you can become an organ and tissue donor. Old age or a history of disease does not mean you can't donate. Organs and tissues that can't be used for transplants are often used to help scientists find cures for serious illnesses.

Many organs and tissues can be donated. The heart, lungs, liver, kidneys and pancreas as well as corneas, bone, skin, heart valves and blood vessels are some of the organs and tissues that can be used to help improve the quality of life for people needing transplants and other surgical procedures.

Signing a donor card will not affect the care you receive at the hospital. If you are injured and brought to an emergency room, you will receive the best possible care, whether or not you have signed a donor card. Donation procedures begin only after all efforts to save your life have been exhausted, and death has been declared.

The miracle of organ and tissue transplantation, each year, saves or greatly improves the lives of thousands of men, women and children. In fact, transplantation is one of modern medicine's greatest triumphs. The true heroes, the miracle makers, are the donors who give the Gift of Life.

Local News: Looking back over the year, it was unbelievable what all we had been through. Although we had a long, hard stressful one, we still had a lot to be thankful for. We had a lot of surprises, good and bad, with still more to come...

It was the Sunday after Christmas on December 29, 1996, when we heard the news. The sun was shining bright – warming a bitter cold day. Although the weather was cheerful enough for late December, I was feeling letdown from all the hustle and bustle from the Christmas holiday. With four adult children and their spouses to shop and buy for, as well as six grandchildren, plus, siblings and friends, it had been a busy one.

While I was making our bed that morning, a knock came at the back door. "Come on in!" Vic called out from the living room. I had no idea to whom it was, but upon hearing all the excitement going on, I didn't waste anytime finding out. It was Alan Murphy, whose parent's lived next door to us. Alan grew up in the neighborhood with our kids, and when marrying, he had moved to the Dale City area just a few miles from us.

"I was just telling Vic," he said, as I walked into the room, "what a good article that was on Doug and Laura in the newspaper."

"It's in the paper!" I exclaimed.

"Yeah," he said. "It's on the front page of the Potomac News! They made top headline, reading, Sister Gives Brother Gift Of Life. They even have pictures of them in color too!"

Knowing we were to be notified a few days prior to its release, we were shocked and flabbergasted about hearing this. And of all days, we had never received our Sunday paper! With it being nine months since the interview with Larisa, we were completely surprised by it all. Having called her two weeks after the interview as to why it was not printed, when told it would be out within a week, she had informed us they were waiting for a special time to print it. Then as the months went by and not hearing from her, we just forgot about it, thinking, it wasn't going to be printed at all. In fact, we wondered at times if we had said or done something wrong to why it wasn't printed.

Alan could not believe we did not get any notice prior to the article's release, or even received the newspaper that day. "I'll get you a newspaper," he said. "Where's your phone?" Alan's son, Nathan, delivered the newspaper in their area, so Alan knew just who to call. After his call, I notified our immediate family to see if they had seen the article yet, which none had. However, having found out, it did not take long for all to round up one. Thanks to Alan, shortly after his call to Potomac News, we had received our paper along with a few extra, as well as being given a humble apology.

When the paper arrived, we could hardly wait to read it. On the front page in big bold headline, read, **Sister gives brother gift of life.** Under the headline was a large color picture of Doug pushing Melissa in her swing in their backyard. Across from that was a picture of Doug sitting, with Laura bending behind him hugging his neck, as well as another smaller picture of Doug by himself.

On the back page was a large 6 by 8 black and white picture of Doug's racing pictures on his rec-room wall, which caption read: **Doug Tuck's memories of capturing stock-car racing championships now grace a wall in his home. He can no longer participate in the sport because of the possibility of injury to the kidney he received from his sister in a February transplant operation.**

With all information true when given for the interview nine months prior, Doug was devastated to what the caption read. He did not want anyone to know he would never be able to race again. But now that he was feeling better, just maybe, he thought, he could go back to racing if he could get Laura and the doctor's approval.

Larisa had done her homework. She did a good job on the article, just as Alan said. She took all the facts and placed them all in the right order, other than Laura's returning to work. Going back seven weeks later, instead of a week that was stated. The article was extremely informative. Ranging from the time of Doug's transplant back to when he was first diagnosed as a diabetic. Larisa issued knowledge on donor organ transplants, along with statements given by Doug's doctors, Jonsson and Shaver, as well as Doug, Sharon, Laura and myself.

"I've always felt like his protector," Laura said in the article. "It broke my heart to see him on dialysis. I feel so fortunate to be healthy enough to help him." "He promised me free oil changes for the rest of his life," she added, laughing at the time of the interview. Dr. Jonsson lamented there are not more living donors like Laura. "It takes a lot of guts ... Praise is in order." he had said.

Larisa summed up the article by informing Doug was an avid stock-car racer, who had won several championships and enough trophies to fill a room. Saying that he had to give up the hobby to avoid the risk of injuring his kidney. In exchange for the thrill of speeding along the track, she further stated, he can now go to the refrigerator whenever he wants to get a drink or a citrus fruit, which was forbidden before the surgery.

"You only live once," Doug said, ending the article. "Race cars are just a piece of metal," he added, referring about not being able to race to Larisa that day while pushing Melissa in her swing.

Searching For Sponsorship: In September 1996, three months before the article appeared in the newspaper, Doug had already begun searching for sponsorship. Even though the first six months of his transplant were pure hell, racing still clung heavy on his mind. Having felt better in seven months time, he received permission from Laura and his doctors to race. He could not wait to get started. To be able to race the following year, he knew he had to find a sponsor.

Knowing his interest with racing, Doug asked Dr. Shaver during one of his appointment visits, "Why don't you sponsor me a race car? You make a lot of money. Look at all the money you made on me!" he told him, laughing. "Just think," Doug said in wanting Dr. Shaver to get a picture of it all, "I could put a big kidney decal on the race car. I'd put Fairfax Transplant Center and your name on it in big letters too," he continued, giving his great sales pitch with lots of enthusiasm.

Doug's sales pitch might have sounded good, but Dr. Shaver didn't buy it. However, he did give him a reference. "Check with Inova," Dr. Shaver told him. "I know the President there. Write, or call to make an appointment with him. I'll even go with you to see him," he added.

Hearing this thrilled Doug. With high hopes, he confronted me to do the letter writing for him. "I hate to ask you Mom," he said, "but could you do a proposal for me to send to Inova Health system? I'd ask

Sharon, but she stays so busy at work and all. I'll never ask you to do another one," he promised.

I had done several racing proposals for Doug in the past. It wasn't the fact that I disliked doing them that bothered me it was the refusals that always came afterwards. I hated seeing Doug get his hopes so high only to be let down each time. It was not only disappointing for him, but for me too.

In writing his proposal to Inova, an innovation of several hospitals in the Northern Virginia area whose mission is to provide quality care and to improve the health of the diverse communities they serve, I wrote it as if Doug had written it. To which, I wrote a one page summary on September 3, 1996. It gave brief statements regarding to whom he was, his medical condition leading up to his transplant, as well as his involvement in racing with past record. Informing, that he would like to pursue his racing with Dr. Shaver giving Inova as a possible sponsor. Saying that employee's, JoAnn Sedlacek and Chris Hartmus, along with others at Fairfax Hospital were intrigued by his racing - backing him 100 percent. It also mentioned, that Dr. Shaver would come with Doug to discuss any further information.

After requesting to please write or call at his (President's) convenience and thanking him for his time and looking forward to hearing from him soon, Doug signed the proposal and mailed it. Like all others in the past, Doug had high hopes getting this sponsorship, whereupon, he anxiously waited for a reply. Although he knew Inova Health System did not need the advertisement, he thought, it would help in other ways. Their logo on his race car, along with awareness on donor-organ transplant, would make people more aware of this much-needed cause. Two long weeks went by before Doug received word. I thought he was going to cry when he read it.

The following was such a reply:

Dated – September 17, 1996
Dear Mr. Tuck:

I was very touched by your incredible story and your new lease on life. I hope you continue to enjoy good health.

We are flattered that you would consider us for sponsorship of your race car.

However, resources in the health field are very restricted at present and we cannot consider your proposal during such tight budgetary times.

I trust you can understand our situation. I wish you luck as you pursue your racing efforts.

Doug's long time dream of ever racing again was shattered. Not because his health this time, but due to not getting sponsorship.

Seeking Job: With Doug doing better by fall, he wanted to find a job. He had been out of work long enough, he thought. Liking his past job installing heat pumps, he knew he would like to continue with something like that. Seeing maintenance workers at Fairfax hospital with past trips, he had mentioned several times he could do that. "I can change light bulbs and do electrical work," he had said, being an all around handy man. "The job would be perfect for you," I told him. "You'd be in doors. Not having to contend with the weather like you did in the past with your old job. It would be great!" Remembering what the social worker had told him prior to his transplant about finding a job, he went to the hospital seeking one.

With him being a transplant patient, he was denied. "There's too many sick people," they told him. "We don't want you catching anything." Doug came home disappointed. "Things aren't working out for me," he said sadly.

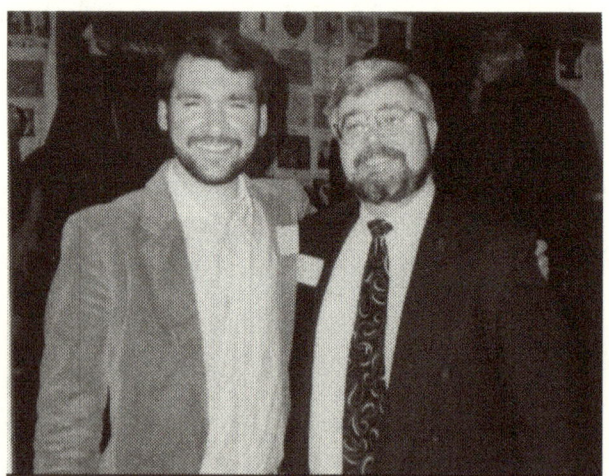

Doug and Dr. Shaver at the
Medal Of Life Ceremony
in Richmond, VA on November 19, 1997.

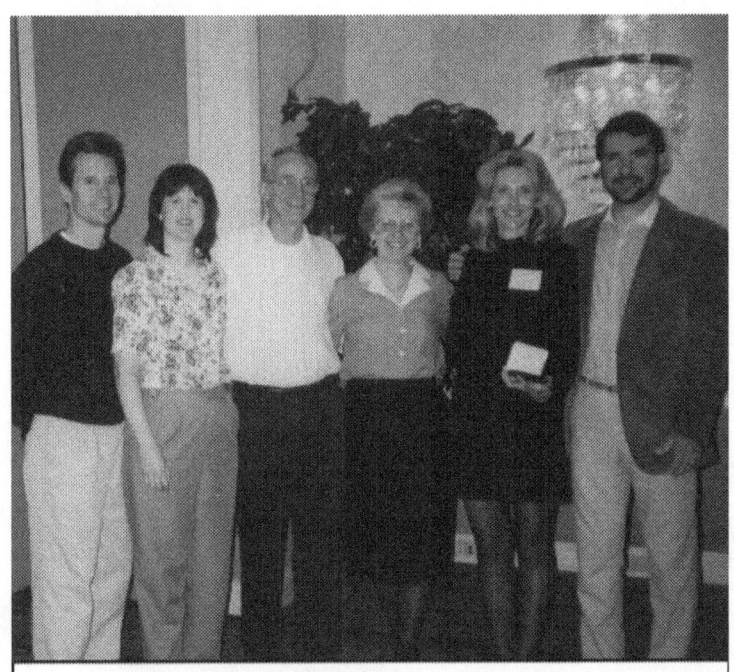

David, Vicky, Vic, Martha, Laura and Doug
in 1997 at the "Medal of Life Ceremony"

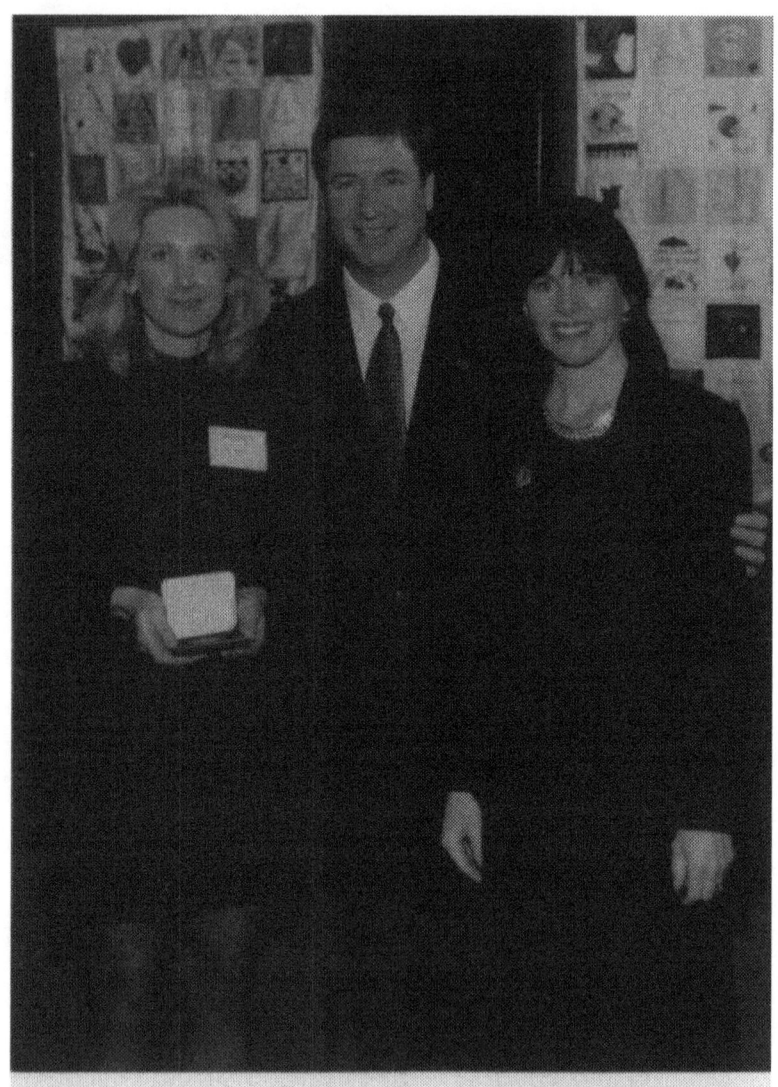

Laura poses with "Medal of Life" award with
Governor George Allen and First Lady.
November 19, 1997

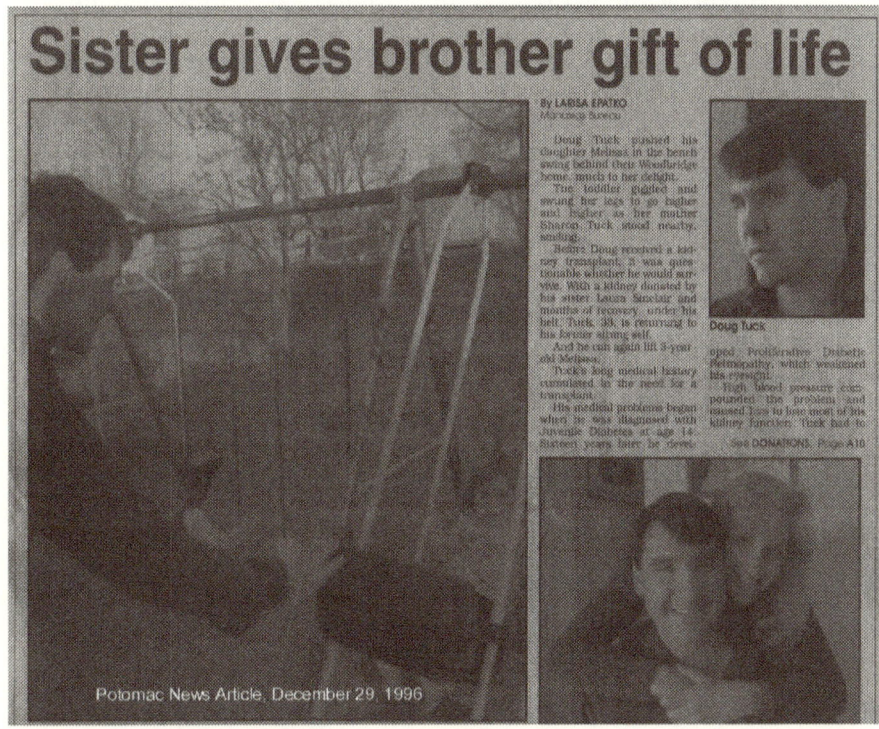

Sister gives brother gift of life

By LARISA EPATKO
Mornings Source

Doug Tuck pushed his daughter Melissa in the bench swing behind their Woodbridge home, much to her delight.

The toddler giggled and swung her legs to go higher and higher as her mother Sharon Tuck stood nearby, smiling.

Before Doug received a kidney transplant, it was questionable whether he would survive. With a kidney donated by his sister Laura Sinclair and months of recovery under his belt, Tuck, 33, is returning to his former strong self.

And he can again lift 3-year old Melissa.

Tuck's long medical history cumulated in the need for a transplant.

His medical problems began when he was diagnosed with Juvenile Diabetes at age 14. Sixteen years later, he developed Proliferative Diabetic Retinopathy, which weakened his eyesight.

High blood pressure compounded the problem and caused him to lose most of his kidney function. Tuck had to

See DONATIONS, Page A10

Doug Tuck

Potomac News Article, December 29, 1996

155

CHAPTER 19

NEW YEAR * NEW BEGINNINGS

Transplant Anniversary: A light snow was falling that mid-afternoon on February 8, 1997, when Doug called Laura to wish her a happy "first" transplant anniversary. Doug had felt lucky to survive that year, which had been a traumatic one for him. One he still talks about but would like to forget. Although he had been doing better in past weeks, he came down with a stomach virus just four days after his first transplant anniversary. Doug was thrilled that he was able to control the situation without being hospitalized.

Having an appointment a month later on March 14 to have a renogram test on his kidney, that gives information regarding function and rate of drainage, he was thrilled no fluid was found and his kidney was doing great. Also having had blood work, he left the hospital that day with a smile, knowing that his creatinine count was 1.8.

Six days later on March 20, we celebrated Doug's 34th birthday – with it much happier than his last. All the stress we had endured was easing some now with him on the road to recovery. However, it didn't last long for there was another crisis to arise in our family. The sudden death of my mother on June 9 with liver cancer, whom just six days prior turned 74. Doug's transplant and Mom's death in fifteen months time was a lot of stress on our family. It was not easy, but somehow we managed to get through those last six months of 1997.

Life Goes On: On February 8, 1998, Doug and Laura celebrated their second transplant anniversary. Health wise, they each were doing well. Although Doug still had good and bad days, we were thankful there were more good ones.

With Doug still on disability and not working, he had kept himself busy by having a full-time job playing Mr. Mom – cooking and taking care of the house. Adding chore, with Melissa, five then, and going to kindergarten, he would take her to and from school as Sharon's work schedule prevented her from doing so. In his spare time, between doctor appointments, he would tend to his vehicles, as well as doing side jobs for family and friends – always staying occupied.

The last six months of the year, though, did not go as well for him. Having had bouts of diarrhea again in June, he was taken off all Cellcept, an immunosuppressive drug, to which the doctor thought might be causing it. With the balance of the drug critical for rejection, he was placed back on it three days later due to a drop of it in his blood work. Whereto, he was told to take one-half the dose he normally took. Having corrected the problem, it was noted the medication probably caused it.

Going back to the hospital for blood work on August 5 and seeing his creainine had went from 1.9 in May up to 2.5, he was told to return the next day for a kidney biopsy. At which time he was stuck six times to get two biopsies. Having another kidney ultrasound as well, he was given great news that good blood flow and no fluid were found.

With the kidney biopsy showing a slight rejection, he returned to the hospital on August 11 to be given his first treatment of 500 units of Solu-medrol, a cortisone drug by IV for one-half hour. The following day he returned for his second treatment, which he was given a half dose and half the treatment time. This did not do anything as his creatinine count went from 2.5 up to 2.7 after treatment. Not given any more treatment, he was sent home with hopes by next appointment his count would be down.

David Turns Forty: The last day of Doug's treatment on August 12, 1998, the family gathered to celebrate David's birthday. As usual, fixing their favorite meal with David's being meatloaf. "No one makes good meatloaf like mom's," he would say.

David was somewhat depressed, having turned forty-years-old, so his Dad and I decided to do something special for him. Thinking it would cheer him up some, we surprised him by having his picture put in our local newspaper. Which a large "bold" caption reading: **Lordy, Lordy, David Tuck is Forty!** When seeing his picture as he leafed through the newspaper that afternoon, he was quite surprised. "That looks just like me!" he later told us when having first glanced at the picture. It did make his day, as he laughed about it several times. Being shocked he said, "Seeing it on the obituary page!"

State Song: Just prior to his birthday, David ran across an article in the newspaper stating that the state of Virginia was searching for a new state song. It was due to a discriminating conflict with "Carry Me Back to Old Virginia," our present one.

Open to the public, songs were to be written and sung with music, then sent in on tape. Not having any singing talents, but well with words, David wrote a song entitled "Virginia Pride." Whereupon, he mailed it to Margie's uncle, Jim Lowery in Texas, who plays bass for a bluegrass band called Saltgrass. Jim volunteered to write music to David's song, and Jim's son, Jason sang the music. With band members recording it, David sent the song tape to Richmond, Virginia. As well as 339 other songs that were sent that contestants entered, with country music singer and writer, Jimmy Dean, one of them.

There would be no prize money for the song chosen, just fame. "Going down in history would be great," said David, of his venture. "Just to make one of the finalist would make me proud!" The winner was to be announced January 1999, the following year.

David waited four long months to find out his song didn't make one of the finalists. There was so much controversy between the contestants and to the ones that did make it, including Jimmy Dean's, that as of right now there has yet to be a winner announced.

Although dishearten his song was not chosen, David has not given up. Now becoming a hobby, he has written several other songs, which he has sent to several well-known country music artists. With one of his songs called, "Grandpa's Legacy," to whom he wrote about my

Dad, his late, Granddad George. He is hoping one day, someone will recognize his talent and make use of all his outstanding work.

Having had a hard time coping with just turning forty, David's song writing hobby did wonders for him. It gave him an outlet, and change, from everyday routine. Turning forty, and being a diabetic for half those years, played a role with him turning another year older, as it's a constant reminder of what the years may bring. Our lives with diabetes would continue, though, it's something that never goes away. You just learn to live with it day by day.

A Continual Battle: After his last visit to the hospital in August, Doug was now having difficulties with his blood pressure medication. Placed on Inderal, a beta adrenergic blocker, along with three other blood pressure medicines he was taking, became too much for him. Though Inderal worked great along with these to help maintain his blood pressure, we found, it was not a good choice for Diabetics.

One afternoon, I found Doug sitting at the dining room table with his head in his hands. Not answering when spoken to him, I turned to find him in great distress. Doug was confused, and disoriented with sweat running down his arms so much that it left a pool of water on the tablemat. He could literally wring his shirt out after one of these attacks, which was not the first he ever had.

Knowing that Inderal masked low blood sugar, Doug was taken off of it due to the many "horrible" insulin reactions he had. He not only had the misfortune of dealing with all the setbacks with his kidney transplant now, but also having to cope with the management of his blood sugar and blood pressure. It was not easy for him.

What Is Blood Pressure? When your heart contracts (beats), it squeezes blood into the arteries and creates pressure in them. This pressure (blood pressure) causes the blood to flow to all parts of the body. Without circulating blood, your organs can't get the oxygen and food they need from your blood to keep functioning. A person's blood pressure constantly changes according to the body's needs. For example, blood pressure will rise during exercise and drop during rest or sleep.

Each time your heart contracts and sends a surge of blood through your arteries, your blood pressure increases. When your heart relaxes between beats, your blood pressure decreases. Because of this, you really have two levels of blood pressure: an upper one when your heart is beating and a lower one when your heart is resting. The higher reading is called the systolic pressure, and the lower one is the diastolic pressure.

Normal blood pressure rises steadily from about 90/60 at birth to about 120/80 in a healthy adult. While there is no ideal number for everyone, the American Health Association considers blood pressure of 120 over 80 to be optimal. When your blood pressure reaches levels above 140 over 90 and stays there, you have what's called high blood pressure, or hypertension. Consistently high blood pressure forces the heart to work far beyond its capacity.

Two Types: There are actually two types of high blood pressure, essential hypertension and secondary hypertension. In essential hypertension, you have raised blood pressure for no apparent reason. In secondary hypertension, your physician has identified the cause of the disorder.

Essential hypertension is more common than secondary hypertension. A tendency toward essential hypertension seems to run in families. In other words, blood pressure appears to be influenced by heredity as well as by life style.

When Doug was first diagnosed with high blood pressure, his reading was 155 over 90. However, when he was a dialysis patient, as well as after his transplant, his blood pressure would rise as high as 185 over 110. Hypertension is often called "the silent killer" because it rarely exhibits symptoms, except for in Doug's case. Throbbing behind his eyes was always a warning signal for him.

By January 1999, Doug's creatinine had stabilized to 2.5. At which time, he was taken off one of his prograf pills – an immunosuppressive drug. With his third transplant anniversary coming up, he was not as lucky as some transplant patients. Having a strong immune system, he had to take twice the anti-rejection medication that most transplant patients never have to do.

Insulin Pump: Being a "brittle" diabetic, David continued having "highs" and "lows" with his blood sugar in spite of doing everything right. A diabetic for 20 years, and seeing his glycohemoglobin (long-term glucose control) count go up, he knew he had to do something about it. Aware that improved blood sugar control would decrease the rate of long-term complications, David invested in an Insulin Pump in February 1999. With proper training on his own, David started using his pump in late March.

Unlike a multiple injection regime, the insulin pump requires fewer injections with a needle, and more freedom to eat at different times of the day. This allows you to control how and when your insulin is delivered so you no longer have to schedule your life around when your insulin is going to work.

Insulin pumps are small, battery-powered devices about the size of a small cell phone or a beeper, that is, about 3 inches by 2 inches by less than 1 inch. They generally weigh 2 to 3 ounces. They can be clipped to your belt or carried in a pocket. Many women discreetly slip the pump into their bra.

The pump connects to you by a thin plastic tube and a soft, flexible catheter, which you implant just beneath your skin and tape in place. This tube-and-catheter combination is known as an infusion set. You can choose your own infusion site; likely spots are the abdomen, the upper part of the outer thigh, or the back of the hip. Your infusion site must be changed every two or three days, as a precaution against infection.

The pump does not automatically know how much insulin to give you. Before each meal and snack, you must test your sugar, decide how many carbohydrates you plan to eat, and then that allows you to tell the pump how fast acting insulin to administer. Also, you must program the machine to administer the basal insulin rates.

There are differences of opinion on who should try the pump. Mature people who are very compliant about their diabetes care, who can take 5-10 blood sugars a day, stay on a strict carbohydrate diet and who are not able to obtain a good glycohemoglobin on conventional therapy should consider intensive therapy.

When David first started using his pump, he overlooked the idea of having to stick himself in the stomach. Something he had never done with past injections. Accepting this now, in knowing, he would only have to do this once every 3 to 4 days. Overjoyed as well, by not having injections everyday as in the past.

First starting on the pump, David had to prick his fingers as much as 20 times per day to keep check on his blood sugar. The most difficult thing he had to deal with was inserting the needle at an angle into his abdomen. With it being painful, he was told about a numbing antiseptic cream, that he now applies to the site an hour before. It was all an experience for him, but he has found that it did wonders for him and his blood sugar control. "It saved my life," he says.

David and his Grandad George in 1959, for whom he wrote the song "Grandpa's Legacy".

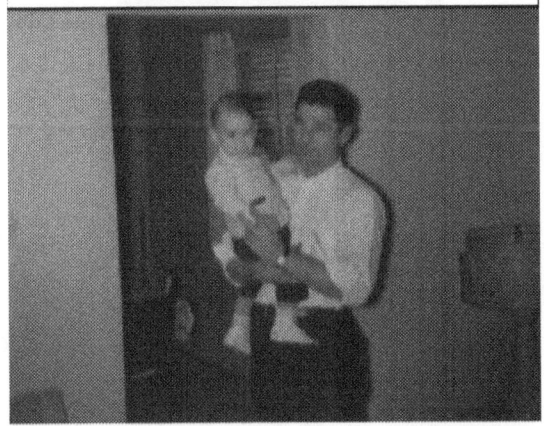

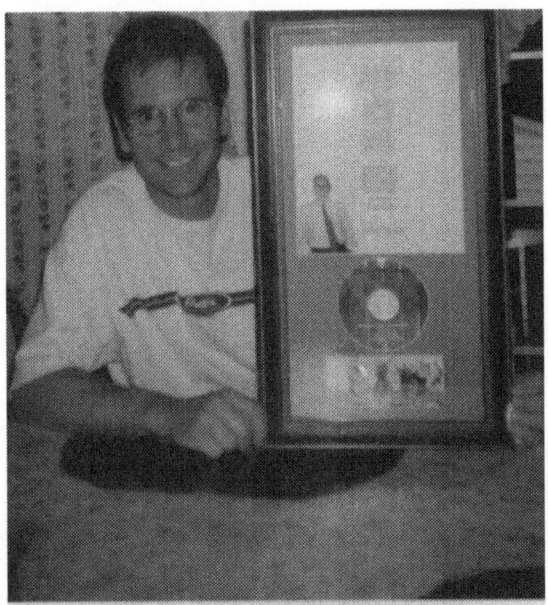

David with framed lyrics and CD of "Grandpa's Legacy" that was recorded and performed by The Saltgrass Band from Texas, written in memory of his late Grandad George.

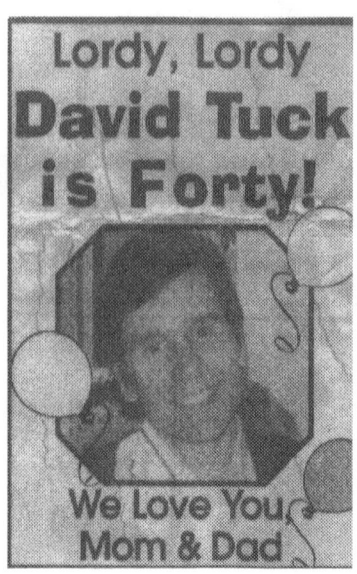

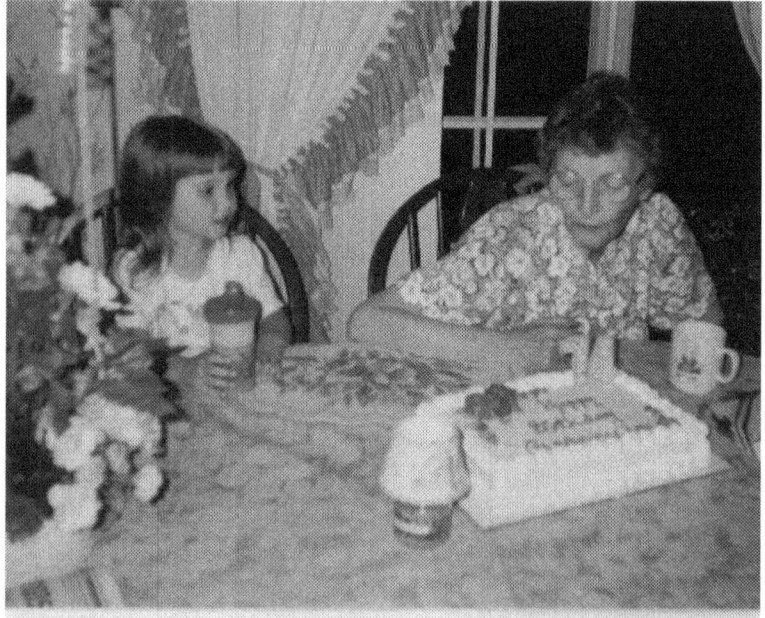

Four-year old Melissa looks on as my mom, Catherine (Eloise) George blows out her 74th Birthday candles on June 3, 1997, just six days before her unexpected death.

CHAPTER 20

ISLET CELL TRANSPLANTS
*
NIGHT OF PURE HELL

Wanting A Cure: Although David's Insulin pump was working well for him, he wanted to do better, and to him, what better way than be rid of diabetes altogether. Considering this, after reading an article about Islet Cell Transplantation from a research progress report in a magazine called Countdown that's put out by the Juvenile Diabetes Foundation.

After reading about islet cell research in the effort to cure diabetes and wanting volunteers for the clinical trials, David called the National Institute of Health (NIH) in Bethesda, Maryland and made an appointment. Qualifying for the transplant, he enrolled, where he was run through a battery of tests in August 1999.

The following is information that was given to him at such time: Islet cell transplantation involves injecting purified islet cells through a recipient's abdomen and into the liver's portal vein. The purified islet cells (which contain insulin producing beta cells) are obtained from the pancreas of an organ donor. The cells take root in the liver – a seemingly benign environment for them – and begin to function normally, secreting insulin and maintaining near perfect blood sugar control.

The appeal of Islet transplantation is that, unlike whole pancreas transplantation, the procedure does not require major surgery, (the islets are injected in a procedure that takes about 15 minutes) and it poses far fewer risks and potential complications for recipients. However, two primary obstacles stand in the way of islet cell transplantation becoming an effective cure for Type 1 diabetes.

*First, because cadaver donors are currently the only viable source of islet tissue for transplantation, the availability of islet cells is extremely limited. Often two donor pancreases are required to generate enough islet tissue for single islet cell transplantation. Moreover, standardized worldwide protocols must be developed to assure that all islets in clinical trials are prepared under the same condition.

*Second, transplanted islets (like all transplanted tissues and organs) are vulnerable to immune system rejection. In addition, the same autoimmune destruction that causes Type 1 diabetes in the first place can attack and destroy the transplanted islet cells.

While sophisticated and highly effective immunosuppressive therapies currently exist to counter the immune attack against transplanted tissues, these agents also reduce the immune system's protective responses, which increase a recipient's risk of infection and disease. Many immunosuppressive drugs have also proven toxic to transplanted islets, and often cause diabetic reactions.

Finding out that islet-cell recipients would need immunosuppressive drugs for the rest of their lives, instead of a short period of time as thought, David decided against the transplant. Although he had all the testing and was given the go-ahead for the transplant, he felt the risk of taking these drugs for the rest of his life was too immense to follow through. His entire immune system would be inhibited, which would leave him vulnerable to other diseases and infections.

Not finding this out until all testing was completed left him disappointed and agitated. It destroyed his hopes of being cured of the devastating disease that he had to deal with for so many years. His only hope then, was that someday, they will be able to create an unlimited supply of genetically engineered beta cells so that successful transplantation can be achieved without the need of immunosuppressive drugs. "Maybe someday," David says hopefully, still displaying the 1990's "Decade for the Cure" magnet on his refrigerator door.

Another Surgery: Around the time David first started using his insulin pump, Doug developed numbness in his right hand. Having pain along with the numbness, he went to the doctor to have it checked out in late August. Diagnosed with Carpal Tunnel Syndrome, which did not get better with treatment, he underwent surgery in November. The doctor claims diabetes may have played a role in some of the damage. Adding another scar, Doug had commented he was beginning to feel like the bionic man.

Night Of Pure Hell: Nearly four months after his hand surgery, Doug went to see Dr. Khosro Shareghi, a Cardiologist, on December 14. For a cardiac evaluation due to chest pain and palpitation, as well as skipped heartbeats he had been having. Seeing large T-waves on his electrocardiogram, suggestive of hyperkalemia (excessive amounts of potassium in the blood), Doug was told by the doctor to go to the Potomac Hospital emergency room for blood testing and treatment. "It was a night of pure hell," Doug would later say.

The blood test showed Doug's potassium level at 5.7, and with normal levels being 3.5 – 5.3, the attending physician was going to call Doug's kidney doctor to relay the information, but Doug insisted he call the transplant center instead.

Dr. Shaver at the transplant center told the physician with Doug having had his transplant for nearly four years, that he would have to get in touch with his nephrologists. Dr. Greenspan was off that day, so the relief doctor gave orders for Doug to have 22 units of regular insulin. Why that much insulin? We do not know!

Knowing his blood sugar was not that high to begin with, Doug did not want the treatment for fear of that much insulin. Even though he stressed his concern, the insulin was given to him anyway. He was also given some brown, nasty, tasting medicine to make him have a bowel movement, saying that this would help bring his potassium level down.

When asking Doug questions while taking his blood sugar, the doctor became concerned when Doug answered through slurred words. At which time, Doug felt his body leaving him. The last thing he heard was the doctor calling out a code alert. Coming to, he saw a swarm of activity, with doctors and nurses racing in and out.

To recover, he was injected with 1600 units of glucose to revive him from a 27 blood glucose reading. Having to stay overnight, he was placed in a room three doors up from where his Granny George passed away just two years prior.

From anxiety due to the procedure, and to which he thought should not have taken place at all, his blood pressure soared to 220 over 110. "My potassium wasn't that high to begin with," he said, upset that he was admitted. "They almost killed me!" Doug was released from the hospital the next morning with a potassium level of 4.6, happy that he had survived!

Cardiologist: Scheduled for a stress test, sonogram, and a 24-hour heart monitor after this episode, Doug went back to the cardiologist on December 20. After all tests were completed and reviewed, the doctor found that Doug had a heart murmur; two leaky heart valves, and fat on his heart. Also finding a left atrial (auricular) muscle enlargement when an echocardiogram was ran, led the doctor to believe Doug might have a heart condition called Hypertrophic Cardiomyopathy. In a severe case, it's a disorder that would obstruct the flow of blood into and out of your heart.

Although the findings were disturbing, the doctor did not think there was anything to be alarmed about. He told Doug that he believed his chest pains were noncardiac. However, in getting a second opinion regarding hypertrophic cardiomyopathy, he was told if chest pains continued he should have further cardiac evaluation at the National

Institutes of Health. Doug was advised to return in six months for a cardiac follow-up.

Doug worried about his heart. He knew the dangers of diabetes and blood pressure, and what damage it could do. "It's taken my eyes and kidneys," he said, after his transplant. "Guess it'll by my heart next." "All I want in life," he says, "is to see my daughter grow up."

Entering the new millennium year all seemed to be going well. David's diabetes was in good control with the use of his insulin pump, and though Doug had been through a lot, more than average, he has come a long way since his transplant in '96. We are thrilled that his creatinine stays in the low twos.

CHAPTER 21

SECOND OPINION * A DREAM COME TRUE

Second Opinion: Wanting to get a second opinion concerning his heart, Doug made an appointment to see Dr. Robert Cunnion, located in Fairfax, Virginia. After a lengthy discussion, Dr. Cunnion decided to run his own tests to rule out Doug having hypertrophic cardiomyopathy. He thought it was unlikely with it an uncommon disorder. "Blood pressure may have caused the enlargement (thickness) to your heart," he informed. Saying that after tests, he would be able to tell Doug more.

To our surprise, Dr. Cunnion had been a past resident of National Institutes of Health for sixteen years, so we knew that he would know just what to look for. Having tests on March 8 and going back on March 19 for test results, Doug and I were overwhelmed with joy to what he had to say. "Your heart is fine!" he told Doug. Doctor Cunnion said with Doug being a diabetic with blood pressure and a kidney transplant, he did excellent on his stress test. "There's few twenty-year-olds in good health could do as well as you did," he commented. "If I had to score you other than number," he added, "I'd place you as a number one athlete." Doug smiled big, knowing he was in such good shape, and his heart was fine.

When asked what numbers one through eight he could do on the treadmill the day of his test, he could tell by the doctor's and the attending assistants' expressions that there's no way, when he told them an eight. Having exercised on an incline for several minutes, he knew he had done well. With Doug and Sharon having a treadmill at home, he was used to this type of exercise. To keep himself in top shape, he would use it when the weather was bad, when he couldn't take his three-mile walks.

Concern With Minioxidil: We were also given the good news that Doug did not have any heart disease. Which ruled out hypertrophic cardiomyopathy. The murmur, leaky valves, and fat found on his heart were found to be of little concern. However, the doctor was concerned about Doug's blood pressure and his taking Minoxidil, one of the strongest blood pressure medicines one can take. It is prescribed for severe high blood pressure not controllable with other drugs. Its natural, expected, and unavoidable drug actions are increased heart rate, fluid retention with weight gain, and excessive hair growth on face, arms, legs and back. Its treatment is not only for high blood pressure, but it also is used to stimulate hair growth as well. The exact mechanism by which this drug stimulates hair growth is not completely known.

Dr. Greenspan placed Doug on minoxidil when he first started dialysis. At one given time, he was taking as much as 32 milligrams a day, considered then, a very large dose. Out of all Doug's medications he hated minioxidil the most. Retaining fluid being one of its side effects is what he said, caused his ankles to swell. With other effects causing darkening of the skin and coarse facial features, and also changing his medium brown hair to black, had changed his appearance somewhat. So much so, that few people recognized him after his transplant.

Doug was taking three other types of blood pressure medications along with the minioxidil. With his blood pressure harder to control after the transplant, it was needed, as a lot of the medication caused increased blood pressure. Even though Doug's blood pressure was 130 over 70 when taken at Dr. Cunnion's office, the doctor's main concern with all his testing was Doug becoming immune to minoxidil. "If it stops working for you," he told him, with it the strongest, "there isn't another drug that can take its place."

After telling Doctor Cunnion about a reliable source that told us old kidneys left during the transplant could cause blood pressure, the doctor suggested they could be surgically removed. He acknowledged even though the kidneys were not working and probably shrunk, they could still be producing a harmful hormone. "I'll talk to your nephrologists about it," he said.

It is funny how fast one can forget about pain. The thought of having surgery after all he'd been through did not faze Doug. He had already checked about having a pancreas transplant, after the diabetic doctor told him he wasn't a candidate for an insulin pump. "You're already in good control," the doctor told him, knowing his hemoglobin A1c count was good, (an indicator that serves as a useful clinical measure of blood sugar control over a long period of time) but not aware of what he had to go through to keep it there.

It was a constant battle for Doug to maintain his blood sugar due to the "highs" and "lows," with most of it caused by his medication. Some days he would have to take five or six shots to bring his sugar down, or it would be the reverse, having to eat more food, and sweets, to help bring his sugar level up. He was tired of it. "How nice it would be," he said, "If I didn't have to deal with that anymore."

On March 20, the day after our seeing Dr. Cunnion, the family gathered that evening to celebrate Doug's 37th birthday. Happy to know his heart test came out all right, and with the fried chicken dinner he ask for, he said it was one of the best birthdays he had in a long time.

True Friend's Knowing his love for racing, friends, Charles and Maryanne Kirtley, approached Doug in late season of '99 to drive their race car. Charles had built the car for his wife, Maryanne, to whom at that time was the only female driver in the Sportsman class. This was the same class that Doug had won championships in. After fulfilling her dream, she gave it up. And out of love and compassion, she and Charles turned the car over to Doug to drive for them.

Being able to race again was a dream come true for Doug. It had been five long years since he'd done so. Racing just four times in the late season of '99, his most gratifying time came in early October when he took the car to Melissa's school for show-and-tell. He was extremely proud that Melissa had told all her first grade classmates her daddy was a race car driver. His chest swelled with pride as he watched Melissa beam as each of her classmates took turns getting into and out of the race car.

Telling us about it later, we could not wait to remind him of what he had said nearly seven-years before when he had found out they were having a girl. "See!" we told him. "You didn't have to have a boy to do all that." Not answering, Doug just smiled from ear to ear.

Championship Blown: Race season of 2000, did not start out well for him. Doug wrecked the first night out, and their sharp looking car was badly damaged. He continued throughout the year, though, without much mishap - running in the top four. The grand finality came in the very last race of the season for the championship, in which the top four runners were contenders. Doug was tied with three others for second place with the leader out by only two points.

The week prior to the last race of the season proved nerve racking to all involved. Some were said to have gotten little sleep. It was a race much talked about throughout the racing circuit at Old Dominion that week. It was quite unusual having that many running for a championship on one given night.

Tension ran high through the pits and grandstands that Saturday night on September 30, 2000, as drivers, fans, and family members waited anxiously for the race to begin. Finally, around 9:30 the Sportsman class filed out, with it the last "big" race of the night.

Melissa, and her little friends' held her daddy's "big" car number 46 signs, as they stood cheering when Doug's name was announced.

Inverting the field to point standings, Doug would be starting third. He was behind number 17, the sixth placed car that had pole position. Tension rose higher as they followed the pace car taking their warm-up laps. As soon as the green flag dropped, we the family knew, Doug had a bad start.

"What's the matter with seventeen?" Vicky yells, as Doug, her brother is held up behind him when taking the green flag. "He's never gone that slow before! He's deliberately holding him back!" she cried out.

Things did not get any better. By the time Doug got around to run with the front leaders, he was taken out on the sixth lap going into turn one. Having the car too beat and not able to continue, devastated Doug. Along with the rest of us – our hearts sank. His chance of winning a championship was gone. Glancing at Melissa with her lip pouted and holding her daddy's sign close to her heart, tears filled her big, brown eyes. Not because he was put out, but thinking her daddy had been hurt.

"I just know I could've won!" Doug told us after the race. Being taken out is something to this day he has not gotten over. With the 2000 racing season over with, he has begun planning for next year. He looks forward to race season 2001, as car owner's Charles and Maryanne will have bought themselves a late-model stock car. Given to Doug to drive, out of "love" for his, and their racing. Doug's dream of driving a late model is finally coming true after fourteen years of waiting. "A few years back," he recalled, "I thought it would never be possible."

Although looking ahead, he still thinks on the past - remembering and recollecting all the good and the bad. Not only with his racing, but health wise too. Due to his sister, Laura, for her unconditional love, he is thankful for all he can still do.

Remembering:

After having checked his blood sugar before climbing into the race car each racing week, he straps himself in. Looking through the lexan windshield at the dark, black asphalt before him with the engine roaring beneath, his sights on victory. Like his diabetes, a challenge he knows he can beat.

Having won two races in the year of 2000, adding to his previous thirty wins at Old Dominion, he smiles proudly. Looking back to the times he has stood in the winner's circle with flag in hand, and as friends and family gathered around him, he looks toward heaven with the bright stars in the sky, and thinks, "Thank you Lord for who I am."

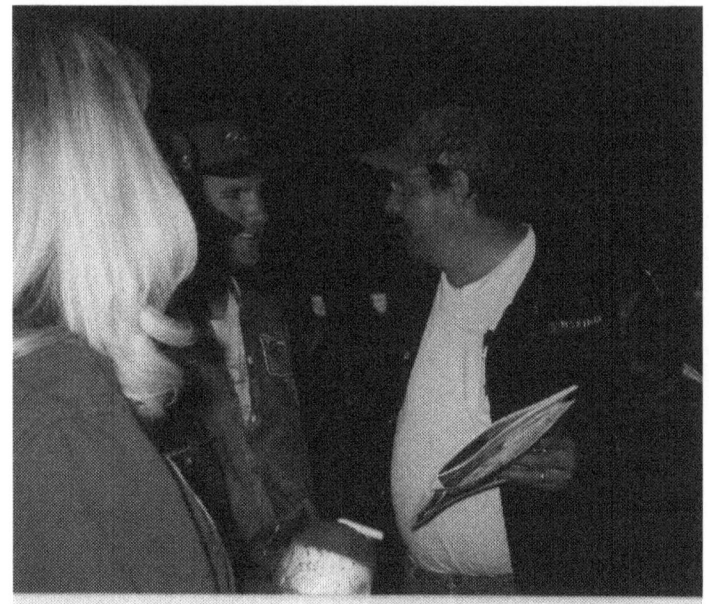

Car #46 owner Charles Kirtley discusses point standings as stated in the Tracks Magazine with Doug as sister Laura looks on.

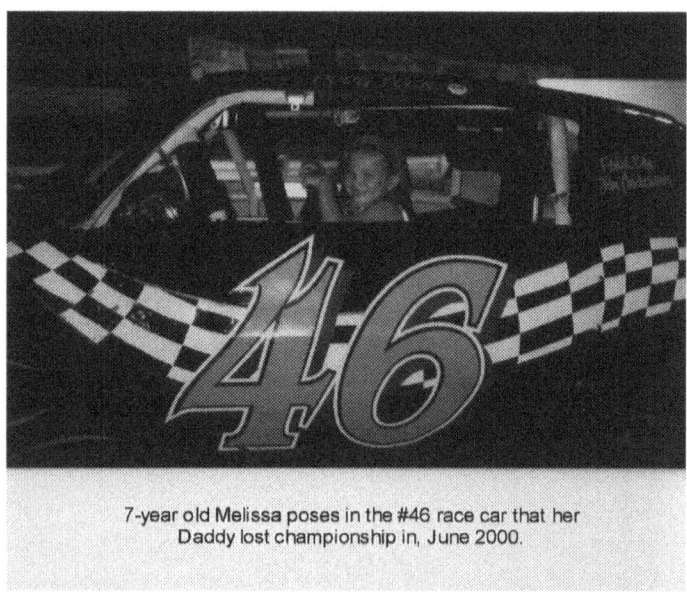

7-year old Melissa poses in the #46 race car that her Daddy lost championship in, June 2000.

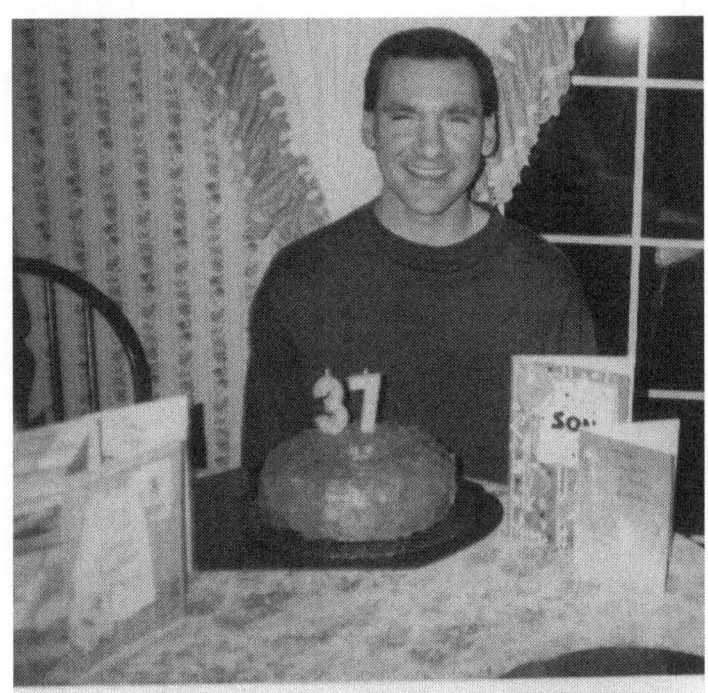

One of Doug's happier birthdays
March 20, 2000

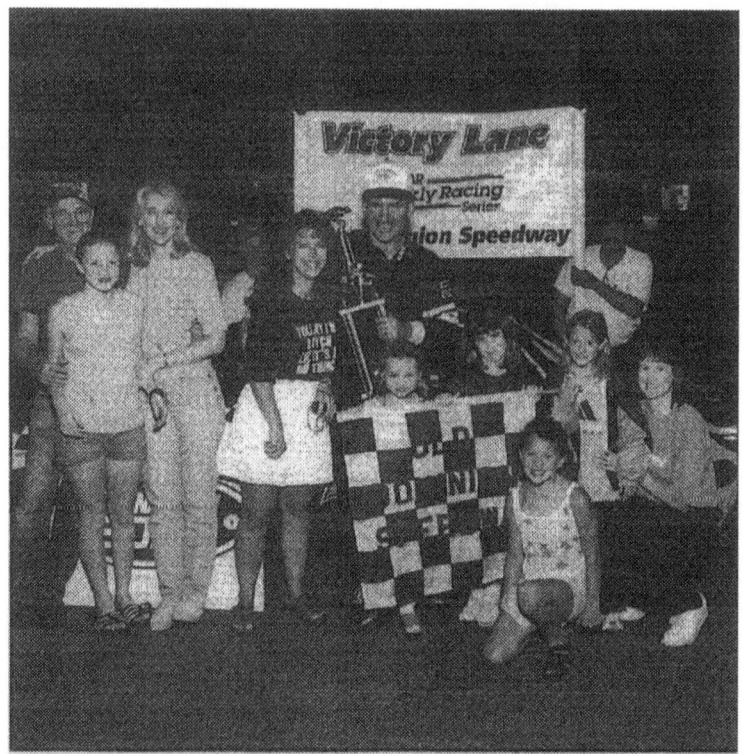

Speedway Sportsman standout Doug Tuck won his second feature event on the season last Saturday. The veteran driver of anything with wheels on it has emerged as the division's newest star...STEVE STEWART PHOTO

Pictured Left to Right:
Dad, Laura, Leah, Sharon, Doug, Melissa (holding checkered flag), friends Britney and Erica, Cari, Vicky and car owner Charles (in background).

CONCLUSION

The moral to my story is sad but true. Diabetes is a disease that can happen to anyone. Researchers believe diabetes is genetically determined and environmentally triggered. Any of us can get diabetes through no fault of our own, virtually any time during our lives. Until researchers unlock the genetic secrets and understand the environmental factors, diabetes will continue to multiply and proliferate. It is a disease that we, as well as the world we live in, will pass on to future generations, unless a cure is discovered.

For people with diabetes, insulin is not a cure but merely a form of "life support". Without insulin, quite simply – they would die. But while insulin allows a person with diabetes to stay alive, it does not prevent, nor delay the complications of the disease. That is why I have devoted time and energy into this book, to help educate, and to recognize the importance to why we would want to wipe out this terrible, lifelong, debilitating disease that afflict so many of us throughout the world.

Our Wish: With Vic now retired and after 47-years of marriage, we are now able to enjoy life. The one thing that would make our life complete is if we could live long enough to see our son's and all the diabetics in the world cured of diabetes. How wonderful that would be!

EPILOGUE

Doug at age Forty-two has come a long way in just nine years. His creatinine stays in the high two's. Told by the doctor that his kidney is sick, his creatinine will not get any better. He is presently on the list for a kidney/pancreas transplant, if and when, time is needed. Purchasing an insulin pump, he hopes it will help manage his diabetes in the meantime.

Developing osteoarthritis since his transplant, he's had surgery on his arm and knee. Just another setback, he found, that he'd have to deal with like all others.

Working for Katz Automobile part-time now, he keeps the place in top shape as well as works on cars - the one thing he knows best. As for his racing, he fills in at times for a different car owner when a driver is needed.

Doug, Sharon and Melissa have added another member to their household. A Pomeranian puppy named Tinkerbell. Melissa at 12-years-old still favors her dad, being just like him. By the time she reaches fifteen, she'll have no problem driving as her dad has taught her how to steer a car – with her driving around the neighborhood in his lap since she was three-years-old.

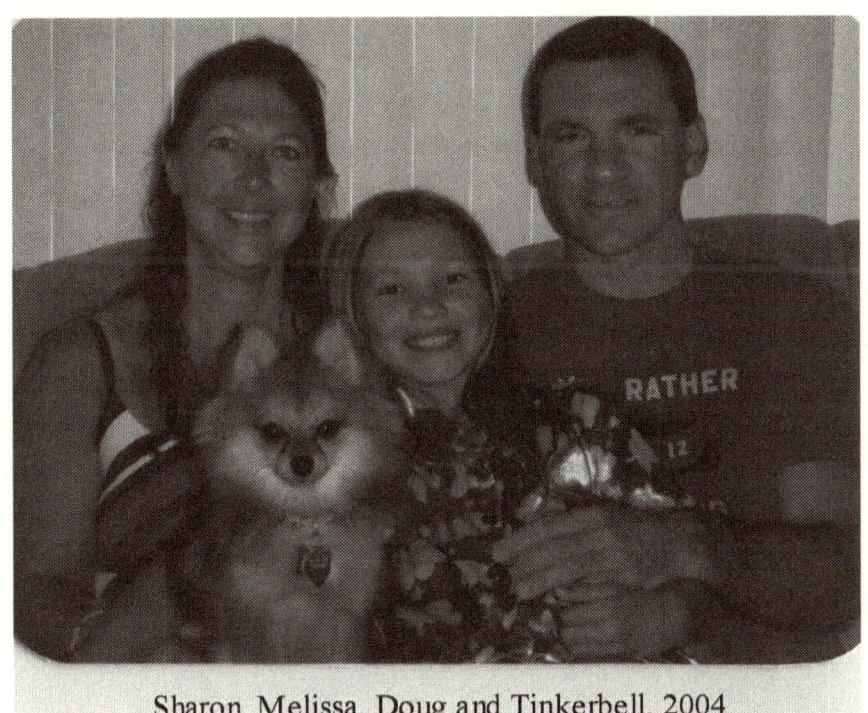

Sharon, Melissa, Doug and Tinkerbell, 2004

David at age 47 continues to do well. Although he still has off days with his blood sugar, he says, "The insulin pump has been my salvation."

Although Jenny 23, and Jessie 21 have left home to pursue their college careers, and working jobs, David and Margie's empty nest was filled with a puppy named Cinda, a sister to Tinkerbell.

David continues to this day writing songs, which some are recorded and played on radio. The most recent that's on CD is written about the love of his life – Margie his wife. A song called "Growing Old With You" that is recorded by the Stevens Family, a Bluegrass band. One of my favorites is called "Grandpa's Legacy" that's recorded by the

Saltgrass Band and is written about my Dad, David's late-Granddad George.

He and Margie celebrated their 25th wedding anniversary on April 5, 2005.

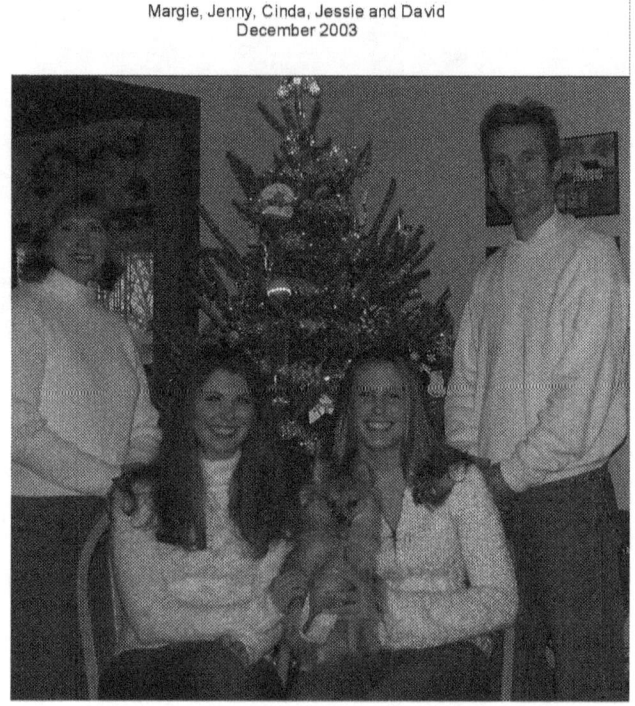

Margie, Jenny, Cinda, Jessie and David
December 2003

Laura at age 43 neither looks nor feels any different than she did 9-years-ago when she became a donor. Finding the man of her dreams, she married Alexander Baker on January 18, 2005. Their lives are richly blessed.

Nearly losing her own life a few years back due to a complicated surgery, she knows what it's like to hold on to life. Giving her incentive to do what she did for her brother, Doug.

Laura's son, Michael 25, and wife, Tanya had a little girl on March 29, 2004, whom they named Alana. Becoming a Grandma has made Laura's life complete.

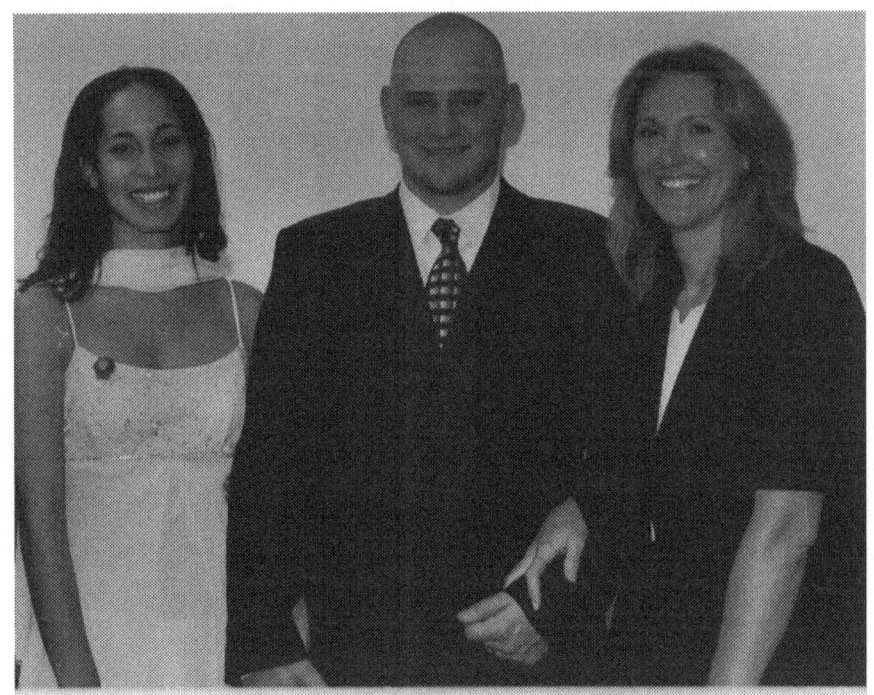

Laura with Michael & Tanya on their Wedding Day
September 28, 2003

Our oldest daughter, Vicky, age 44, that's not mentioned but one time in my memoir, has been there for her brother's and sister, to whom she is very close. Standing by her Dad and me through it all, she was a Godsend.

With her working for the Federal Bureau of Investigation and her husband, William (Willie) as a Capital Policeman, their days are filled with justice.

Daughter's, Leah, at 17, and Cari 14, are involved like most others at this age, school and sports.

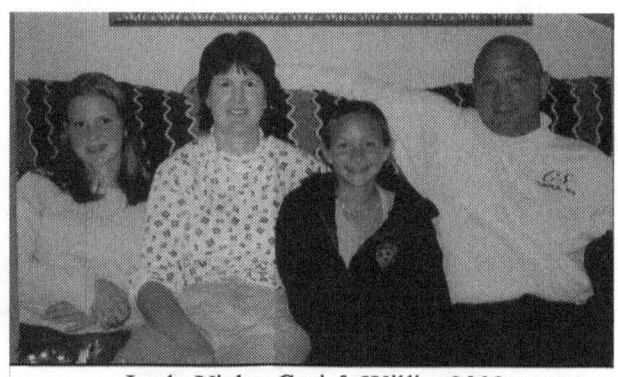

Leah, Vicky, Cari & Willie, 2003

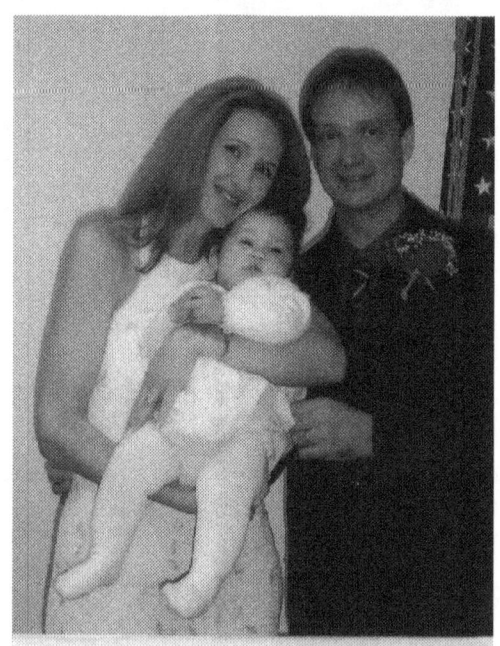

Laura and Alex on their wedding day, with Laura's granddaughter Alana, January 18, 2005.

www.ingramcontent.com/pod-product-compliance
Lightning Source LLC
Chambersburg PA
CBHW031320290526
45784CB00014B/368